MW01526088

Low Oxalate Cookbook

Low Oxalate Diet Cookbook With Nutritional Guide To Prevent Kidney Stones

Laura Evans

Copyright © 2020

All rights reserved. No part of this publication may be reproduced, distributed, or transmitted in any form or by any means, including photocopying, recording, or other electronic or mechanical methods, without the prior written permission of the publisher, except in the case of brief quotations embodied in critical reviews and certain other noncommercial uses permitted by copyright law.

ISBN: 9798614142216

Limit of Liability

The information in this book is solely for informational purposes, not as a medical instruction to replace the advice of your physician or as a replacement for any treatment prescribed by your physician. The author and publisher do not take responsibility for any possible consequences from any treatment, procedure, exercise, dietary modification, action or application of medication which results from reading or following the information contained in this book.

If you are ill or suspect that you have a medical problem, we strongly encourage you to consult your medical, health, or other competent professional before adopting any of the suggestions in this book or drawing inferences from it.

This book and the author's opinions are solely for informational and educational purposes. The author specifically disclaims all responsibility for any liability, loss, or risk, personal or otherwise which is incurred as a consequence, directly or indirectly, of the use and application of any of the contents of this book.

DEDICATION

To All who desire to live And Eat Healthy

TABLE OF CONTENT

INTRODUCTION

What Are Oxalates?

Oxalates are organic molecules present in plants, they occur as an end products of metabolism in series of plant tissues. Oxalates are present in plants and also present in humans in abundance, they work in humans to provide important natural bacteria with required nutrients, hereby serving as pre-biotics. They work in plants to bind with calcium, functioning to keep excess nutrients in check. Too many of these molecules in the body can cause significant complications such as kidney stones. Where too much oxalate is present in the body, oxalates binds with calcium, thus forming a kind of crystal that stays glued together to form stones.

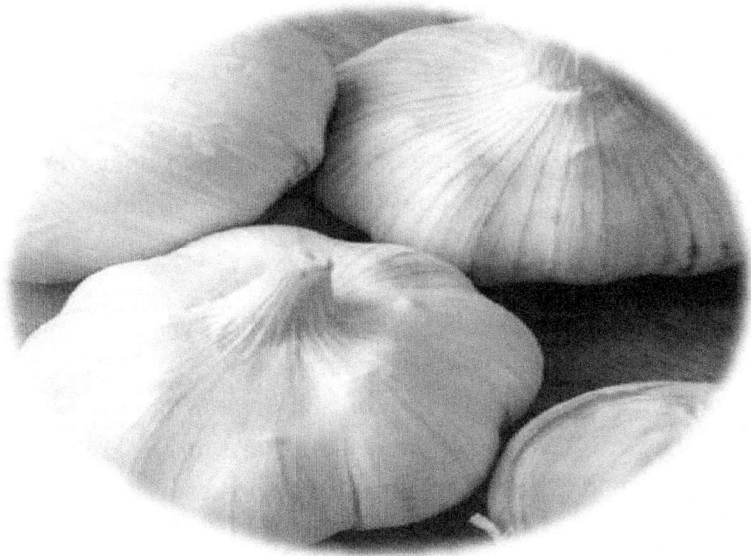

What Is The Relationship Between Oxalates And Kidney Stones

According to National Kidney Foundation, calcium oxalate stones are the most common type of kidney stones.

Kidney stones are a widely known kidney problem. This is a situation where substance and other mineral properties in the blood obstruct the kidneys, forming solid masses (stones). During urination, kidney stones are excreted; they cause severe pain in the abdomen, groin or flank and can lead to many other significant complications.

The usual process is when you consume food with oxalate; they are transported through the esophagus down to the digestive system and are excreted either as stool or urine. But when oxalate present in the body is high, oxalates binds with calcium, thus forming a kind of crystal that stay glued together to form stones. In conclusion, high oxalate level in the body increases the chance of having kidney stones.

Risk Of Having Kidney Stones

These factors can also increase the risk of forming kidney stones

Certain medical conditions, obesity, and history of digestive disorders

Not drinking enough fluid

If you take antibiotics regularly, these antibiotics will make micro-organisms fall which also reduce your defense

High protein in diet or too much salt, and sugar in diet

Although vitamin C is a good source of nutrient for the body but foods too high in vitamin C has proven to increase oxalate levels in the body

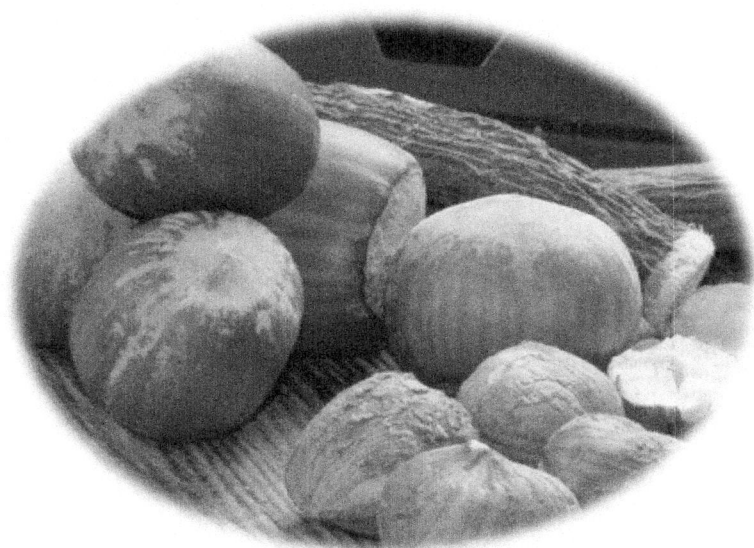

How to control oxalate for kidney stones

Apart from following a low oxalate diet, there are different strategies you can adopt to help reduce oxalates level in your body. Drink lots of fluid (water) on a daily basis to keep calcium oxalates from forming.

It's also beneficial to incorporate calcium into your diet. When calcium in your diet is too low, oxalates in your body will be high and you will be at a higher risk of having of kidney stones.

Reduce the consumption of salt per day; just a little sodium is okay to keep the system functional. You can control the amount of ingredients and spice you use when you prepare your own food.

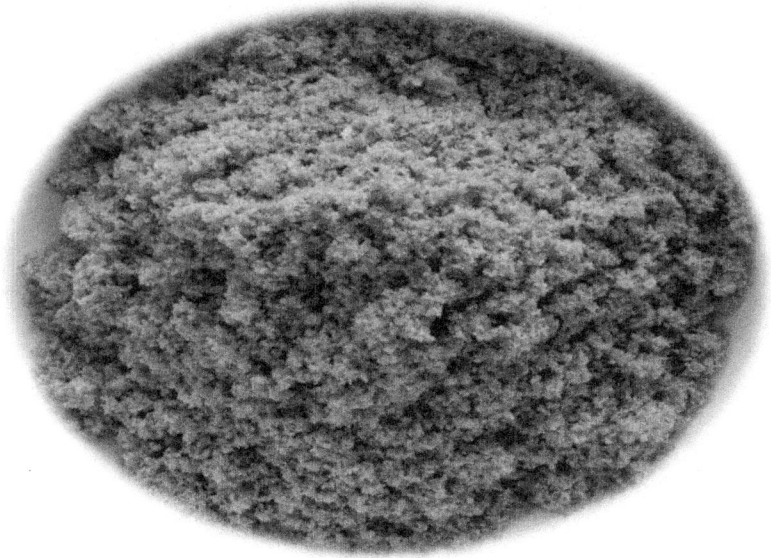

The low-oxalate diet

The best way to avoid kidney stones is by cutting down on the amount of oxalates that you consume; this will make less oxalate present in your intestinal tract for absorption. Although there is no agreement whatsoever on the number of oxalate that are acceptable in low low-oxalate diet. However, according to National Kidney Foundation, it is most reasonable to stick to oxalates below 100 mg per day; best idea is to stay below 50 mg per day.

To achieve this goal, a list of food and oxalates contents was created as a guide on the low oxalate diet and updated by the University of Chicago. The rule is simple, avoid high oxalate foods, and concentrate on food with low oxalate contents.

Who Can Benefit From A Low-Oxalate Diet?

Anyone that has calcium oxalate kidney stones with high urinary oxalate level can benefit from a low-oxalate diet. The reasonable thing to do is switch from your present dietary lifestyle to more suitable low oxalate diet to help reduce any potential risk of another stone from forming.

Practical Steps You Can Take To Control Oxalate For Kidney Stones

1. The key is to eat plenty low oxalate food and few high-oxalate foods.
Eating high oxalate food increases the oxalate that will be available for absorption from your digestive tract.
There is no way you can totally eradicate oxalate from your food, because most plant contain oxalate. The Simple rule is eat healthy but be selective and go more on low oxalate foods combined with calcium rich foods.

2. Reduce the amount of sodium in your diet.
Its important to cut down food with much sodium in your diet, about 2-3 grams per day. You can discuss with a dietitian on how to make changes to your meal plan. Do away from eating packaged foods, they often contain high sodium. Deli meats, dry soup mixes, canned products, hot dog and other processed food may not be a good option of food to eat.

3. Increase your daily Fluid Intake.
Water is very good for the body. It is very important to take about 10-12 glasses of fluid daily; about 5-6 of the fluid should be mainly

water. However, it is considered that lemonade is also beneficial to help reduce the risk of forming calcium oxalate stone.

4. Cut down on vitamin C on your diet.
No doubt vitamin C plays an important role in our nutrition diets. However, high intake of this nutrient may spike-up the level of oxalate in your urine, so the risk of forming calcium oxalate kidney stones is increased.
Oxalate production is an end product of Vitamin C (ascorbic acid) metabolism, anyone taking any amount of Vitamin C more that 500 mg per day may be at risk of kidney stones.

5. Watch out for amount of protein you eat daily.
Consuming too much protein can expose you to high risk of kidney stones. Limit protein to about 4 to 6 ounces per servings a day.

6. Increase the amount of calcium you eat.
You do not need to fret at the mention of calcium, yes eating food rich in calcium can helps reduce the number of oxalate your body will absorbed, so the chances of forming stones is reduced because calcium binds oxalate in the intestines. Low calcium in your diet will put you at the risk of forming calcium oxalate kidney stones.

Easy Steps To Increase Calcium

When calcium in your diet is too low, level of oxalates in your body will be high and you will be at a higher risk of having of kidney stones
Vitamin D helps our body to absorb calcium, so if there is not enough of it, our body won't be able to make good use of the calcium we are eating. Consume more vitamin D.

You can get vitamin D from foods such as Portobello mushrooms, egg yolks, tuna and salmon.

Dairy options like yogurt, milk, cheese and other dairy products

Fruits such as orange juice, blackcurrants, bananas, lemons etc

Add calcium-fortified foods to your grocery list

Oxalate Content Of Foods Lists

Drinks	Oxalate content
Apple Juice	Very low
Apple Cider	Unknown
Buttermilk	Very low
Cranberry Juice	Very low
Coffee (Instant)	Very low
Coffee	Very low
Coconut Milk	Unknown
Club Soda	Unknown
Chocolate Milk	High
Cherry Juice	Low
Decaffeinated Products	Varies
Grapefruit Juice	Very low
Grape Juice-White	Low
Grape Juice-Red	Medium
Grape Juice-Purple	Unknown
Juice from Concentrate	Varies
Milk	Very low
Orange Juice-Frozen	Very low
Orange Juice-Fresh	Very low
Pineapple Juice	Very low

Peppermint Tea	Very low
Rice Milk-Vanilla	Very High
Rice Milk-Carob	Very High
Spearmint Tea	Very low
Soybean Milk	Very High
Tomato Juice (Canned)	Medium
V8 Juice	High

Fruits	Oxalate content
Avocados	Very Low
Apricots-Fresh	Very Low
Apples, Red Delicious	Low
Apples, Jonathan	Low
Apppples, Granny Smith	Low
Apples, Golden Delicious	Low
Blueberries	Unknown
Blackberries	Very High
Bananas	Medium
Custard Apple	Unknown
Currants, Red	High
Currants, Black	High
Cherries-Fresh	Very Low
Cherimoya	Unknown
Casaba (Melon)	Low
Cantaloupe	Unknown

Canned Fruits	Varies
Dewberries	High
Dates	High
Figs-Fresh	Very High
Figs-Dried	Very High
Grapes, Red	Low
Grapes, Green	Very Low
Grapefruit	Unknown
Gooseberries	High
Hucklesberries	Low
Honeydew	Very Low
Jicama	Unknown
Kumquats	Very Low
Kiwifruit	Very High
Lychees	Low
Limes	Medium
Lime Peel	High
Lime Juice	Low
Limes	Medium
Lemon Peel	High
Lemon Juice	Low
Lemons	Very Low
Mangos	Low
Mandarin Oranges	Medium
Necatarines	Unknown
Oranges	High
Orange Peel	High
Prunes	Unknown
Plums	Low

Plantains	Unknown
Pineapple	Low
Perimmons	High
Pears-Unpeeled	Medium
Pears-Peeled	Low
Peaches	Very Low
Passion Fruit	Very Low
Papayas	High
Raspberries, Red	High
Raspberries, Black	Very Low
Raisins	Low
Star Fruit	Very High
Sharifa	Unknown
Tangerines	Unknown
Tamarind	Unknown
Watermelon	Very Low
Grains	Oxalate contents
Amaranth	High
Alfalfa Sprouts Delicious	Low
Bulgar	Unknown
Buckwheat	Very High
Barley	High
Cornstarch	Medium
Corn	Low
Flour (Wheat)	Very High
Durum Flour	Very High

Millet	Very High
Kamut	High
Oats	Medium
Pasta	Varies
Pappadum	Varies
Quinoa	Unknown
Rye	Very High
Rice Flour	Unknown
Rice-White	Very Low
Rice-Brown	Medium
Sprouted Grain Bread	Unknown
Spelt	Unknown
Sorgum Flour	Unknown
Triticale	Unknown
Tapioca	Unknown
Wheat	Very High
Wheat Germ	Unknown

Legumes, Nuts & Seeds	Oxalate Content
Almonds	Very High
Butter Beans	Unknown
Brazil Nuts	Unknown
Black-eyed Peas	Low
Black Beans	Very High
Bean Sprouts	Unknown
Bean Flour	Varies
Coconut	Very Low
Chick Peas	Medium

Chestnuts (canned)	Very Low
Chestnut Flour	Unknown
Cashews	Very High
Coconut Flour	Unknown
Canellini Beans	Unknown
Flax Seed	Low
Filberts (Hazelnuts)	Very High
Faba Beans	Unknown
Garfava Flour	Unknown
Garbanzo Beans	Medium
Kidney Beans	High
Lentils-Boiled	Medium
Mung Beans	Medium
Mung Bean Sprouts	Low
Miso	Unknown
Macadamia Nuts	low
Navy Beans	Very High
Pumpkin Seeds	Medium
Pistachio Nuts	High
Pinto Beans	High
Pine Nuts	Very High
Pecans	Very Low
Peas-Boiled	Very Low
Peanut Butter	Very High
Peanuts	Very High

Pea Flour	Unknown
Split Peas-Yellow	Low
Split Peas-Green	Medium
Soybeans	Very High
Soy	Very High
Sesame Seeds	Very High
Seed Flour	Varies
Seed Butters	Varies
Tofutti Cheese	Unknown
Tofu	Medium
Tahini	Very High
Walnuts	Very High

Meats	Oxalate Content
Anchovies	Unknown
Beef	Neg
Bacon	Neg
Canned Fish	Unknown
Fish	Neg
Eggs	Neg
Hot Dogs	Unknown
Ham	Neg
Lamb	Neg
Meats (Processed)	Unknown
Meats (Canned)	Unknown
Meats	Neg
Pork	Neg
Poultry	Neg
Smoked Meats	Unknown
Shellfish	Neg
Sashimi	Unknown

Baking Ingredients	Oxalate Content
Apple Cider Vinegar	Very Low
Baking Soda	Neg
Baking Powder	Very Low
Baker's Yeast	Medium
Cocoa Powder	Very High
Chocolate	Very High
Cream of Tartar	Very Low

Gelatin (unflavored)	Very Low
Xanthan Gum	Unknown
Vinegar	Low

Condiments	Oxalate Content
Apple Cider Vinegar	Very Low
Ketchup	Very Low
Mayonnaise	Low

Sweeteners	Oxalate Content
Aspartame	Very Low
Corn Syrup	Very Low
Date Sugar	High
Evaporated Cane Juice	Very Low
Granulated Glucose	Unknown
Honey	Very Low
Molasses	Unknown
Maple Syrup	Very Low
Sugar	Very Low
Sucralose	Very Low
Stevia	Very High
Splenda	Very Low
Saccharine	Very Low
Turbinado Sugar	Very Low
Tagatose	Unknown
Xylitol	Unknown

Vegetables	Oxalate Content
Asparagus	Low
Artichokes (French)	Medium
Acorn Squash	Very Low
Bok Choy	Very Low
Beets	Very High
Bitter Gourd	Unknown
Butternut Squash	Unknown
Bamboo Shoots	Unknown
Broccoli Tips-Boiled	Low
Broccoli-Raw	Medium
Brussel's Sprouts-Raw	Medium
Broccoli-Steamed	High
Burdock Root	Unknown
Brussel's Sprouts-Boiled	Low
Broccoli-Boiled	Low
Brussel's Sprouts-Steamed	High
Black Radish	Unknown
Canned Vegetables	Varies
Cucumbers	Very Low
Courgette (Zucchini)	Very Low
Collard Greens-Steamed	High
Collard Greens-Raw	Low
Cabbage-Green-Raw	Low
Carrots-Boiled	Medium
Collard Greens-Boiled	Medium

Cauliflower-Raw	Low
Carrots-Raw	Very High
Cauliflower-Boiled	Very Low
Cauliflower-Steamed	Low
Celeriac-Fresh	Unknown
Celeriac (Canned)	Medium
Celery-Raw	Very High
Chard	Very High
Chickory Root	Unknown
Carrots-Steamed	Very High
Chili Peppers	High
Cabbage-Red	Unknown
Cabbage-Green-Steamed	Medium
Cabbage-Green-Boiled	Low
Dandelion Greens	High
Eggplant	Medium
Green Beans	Very Low
Garlic	Unknown
Haricot Beans	Unknown
Jalapenos	Unknown
Kale	Unknown
Kudzu (Kuzu)	Unknown
Kimchi	Unknown
Lettuce	Very low
Leek	Medium

Mushrooms	Very Low
Onions	Low
Olives-Black	Very High
Olives-Green	Very High
Okra	Very High
Pumpkin-Raw	Neg
Pumpkin-Canned	Very Low
Potatoes-Unpeeled	Very High
Potatoes-Peeled	Very High
Potatoes, Red-Peeled	Medium
Pickles (Dill)	Very Low
Peppers, Red	Very Low
Peppers, Green	Medium
Parsnips	Unknown
Rutabaga	Unknown
Rhubarb	Very High
Radishes, White	Very Low
Radishes, Red	Neg
Sweet Potatoes	Very High
String Beans	Medium
Spinach-Frozen	Very High
Spinach-Fresh	Very High
Spaghetti Squash	Unknown
Sorrel	High
Seaweed	Medium
Sauerkraut	Medium
Turnips	Very Low

Tomatoes-Fresh	Medium
Tomato Sauce-Canned	High
Tomato Puree-Canned	High
Tomato Paste-Canned	High
Taro	Unknown
Watercress	Neg
Water Chestnuts	Very Low
Yucca Root	Unknown
Yams	Unknown
Zucchini	Very Low

OXALATE CONTENT UPDATE

1 teaspoon of Cinnamon contains 38.5 mg oxalate content.
1/4 teaspoon of nutmeg contains 2.3 mg oxalate content
1 tablespoon of olive oil contains 0.9 mg oxalate content
Half cup of chopped onion contains 3.3mg oxalate content
1 clove garlic contains 0.3 mg oxalate content
1 tablespoon of raw ginger, 6.3 mg
1 tablespoon of green chiles contain 2.2 mg oxalate content
Swanson's chicken broth (none),
Cayenne pepper (1.3 mg. per fourth teaspoon), oregano
(1 teaspoon for ground oregano contains 7.3 mg oxalate content
1 tablespoon of lime juice contains about 0.3 mg oxalate content
Half cup of Black-eyed peas contains about 3 mg oxalate content
Fresh cilantro (1.4 per fourth cup),

1 tablespoon of sesame seeds has whopping 196 mg oxalate content

1 tablespoon sesame oil has 0.4 mg.

1/2 cup of Sweet rice flour has about 10.4 mg. oxalate

1/2 cup of cottage cheese has 2.9 mg; Half cup of most cheese is about 2-2.9mg

1/4 cup of coconut flour has about 2.2 mg. oxalate

Eggs, salt and coconut oil are very low oxalate

Half cup of Rolled oats 11.1 mg oxalate

2 tablespoons of Sun butter, 6.1 mg

Half cup of ground flax seed, 6.6 mg

2 tablespoons of pumpkin seeds, 5.2 mg

1 teaspoon of Celtic sea salt about 0.2 mg oxalate

1 garlic clove about 0.3 mg oxalate

Half cup of Asparagus, about 4.9 mg oxalate

1 tablespoon of dill about 10.5 mg oxalate

2 ounces of Ground sausage, about 6.0 mg oxalate

Half cup of boiled collard greens, about 8.7 mg. oxalate

Half cup of Brussels sprouts when boiled for 12 minutes is about 8.5 mg and 12.7 mg when steamed

1 tablespoon of peanut oil, about 0.6 mg oxalate

Half cup of celery, about 7.o mg oxalate

1/2 cup of canned kidney beans, about 7 mg. per and uncooked is about 11.7 mg

1/2 cup coconut milk, about 0.0 mg if using a brand without guar gum Natural Value or Chaokoh

Half cup of Uncle Ben's long grain white rice, about 0.9 mg when boiled

1 teaspoon of thyme, about 2.5 mg oxalate

Sautéed pepper habenero pepper, about 0.4 mg oxalate

Half cup of Big Beef tomato, about 4.2 mg oxalate

Half cup of Early Girl tomato, about 5.9 mg oxalate
Half cup of Brandy Wine, about 4.9 mg. oxalate
2 tbsp of honey (about 0.6mg oxalate
1 tbsp of olive oil (0.9mg oxalate)
1/2 tsp of xanthan gum (unknown mg)
1/4 tsp of baking soda (0 mg)
1/4 tsp of cream of tartar (0.25mg oxalate)
4 tbsp of ground linseed/flax (2.8mg oxalate)
1/4 cup of brown rice flour (14.4mg oxalate)
1 cup of red pepper (about 3.6 mg oxalate)
1 tsp of black pepper (about 12 mg oxalate)

BREAKFAST AND DRINKS

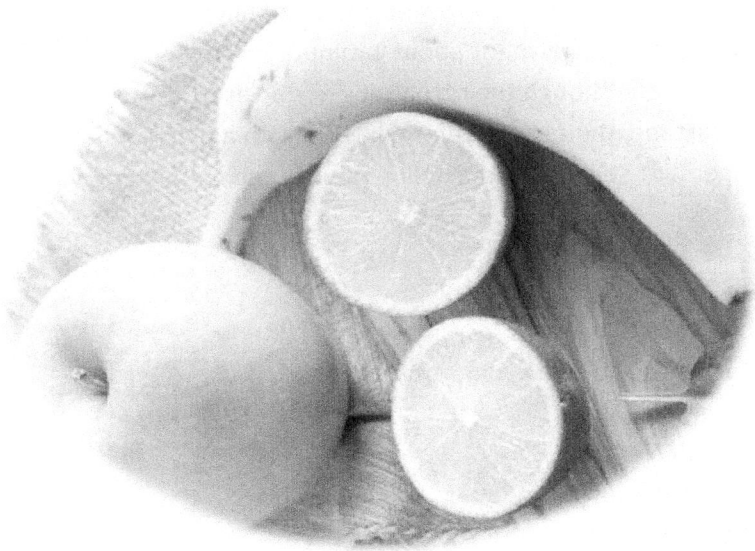

Milky Steamer

Servings: 1-2

INGREDIENTS

1 cup of milk

A dollop of whipped cream

1/4 cup of Torani's sugar free Chocolate Syrup

A pinch of mace or 1 Peppermint stick stirrer

INSTRUCTIONS

1. Use a large measuring glass cup to mix the syrup and milk together until well combined. Run through the steamer attachment on your cappuccino or coffee maker, if you have one.

2. Alternatively, warm for about 1 minute on stove top or in the microwave. Although the result may not be as frothy as it should, but trust me, the taste is yummy! Serve with a pinch of mace or a Peppermint stir stick and a dollop of whipped cream. Enjoy!

Watermelon Ice Cubes

Prep Time: 15 minutes

Total Time: 2hours 15 minutes

Servings: 24 cubes

INGREDIENTS

1 tbsp of lemon juice

1 tbsp of honey

1/2 cup of water

1 1/2 cups watermelon, seeded and cut into medium thick slices

INSTRUCTIONS

1. Combine the entire ingredients to a blender and puree until smooth.

2. Pour puree into ice cube trays and freeze for few hours.

3. Serve in a glass cup of water or lemonade.

Blueberry Banana Milkshakes

Servings: 2

INGREDIENTS

(Optional) 1 tablespoon of honey

1 cup of coconut milk

1/2 cup of frozen blueberries

1 frozen banana

INSTRUCTIONS

1. Blend the banana, coconut milk, blueberries and honey in a blender or food processor until smooth (You can thaw banana for 10-15 minutes if too frozen before adding to the blender in order for it to incorporate with other ingredients. Serve in 2 frosty mugs.

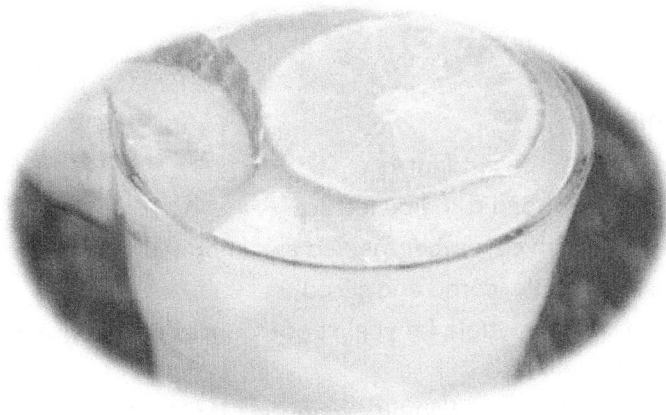

Banana Smoothie

INGREDIENTS

1 ripe banana

1 cup of bok choy 40 g

1 cup of collard greens 30 g

1/2 cup of frozen strawberries 75 g

1 tbsp of raw pumpkin seeds

8 ounces of unsweetened calcium-fortified soy milk

INSTRUCTIONS

1. Combine the entire ingredients in a blender and blend until smooth and creamy.

Lime Cucumber Smoothie

Prep Time: 10 minutes

Cook Time: 15 minutes

Servings: 2

INGREDIENTS

(Optional) 1 – 5 sprigs cilantro

1 – 2 cup of chopped romaine lettuce

1 medium English cucumber, peeled and chopped

1 Fuji or Gala apple, cored and sliced

10 ounces of plain whole fat yogurt or 8 ounces of coconut milk

Juice of 1 small lime

(Optional) 2 teaspoon of liquid coconut oil (MCT oil)

2 tablespoons of flax seed, (sprouted is best)

INSTRUCTIONS

1. Combine the entire ingredients in a blender and blend until smooth and creamy. Let sit for at least 5 minutes before serving.

Red Peppers Stuffing

Prep Time: 15 minutes

Cook Time: 60 minutes

Servings: 2-3 servings (10.3 mg)

INGREDIENTS

(Optional) Fresh thyme sprigs for garnish

6 medium red bell peppers, cut tops and hollowed off

1/2 cup of pumpkin seeds

1/2 cup of dried cranberries

1 tsp of white pepper

1/2 tsp of salt (or to taste)

2 Granny Smith apples, peeled and diced finely (1 1/2 cups)

1 cup of diced onions

1/2 cup of diced celery

2 tbsp of olive oil

1 tsp of dried sage

2 tsp of dried thyme

1 cup of long grain white rice

1 cup of apple cider

1 fennel seed tea bag

INSTRUCTIONS

1. Heat-up the oven to 350 F.

2. Add apple cider and 1 cup of water to a medium saucepan and bring to a boil. Add the tea bag and brew for at least 5 minutes, then remove.

3. Add in rice, sage and thyme. Cook covered and return to boil. Simmer for about 20 minutes until all liquid is absorbed.

4. While the rice is cooking, heat olive oil over medium heat in a large skillet. Add onions, celery , apples, pepper and salt and sauté for about five minutes.

5. Combine the sautéed vegetables, cooked rice and fruit. Stir in the pumpkin seeds and cranberries.

6. Fill the bell peppers with the stuffing, then place the stuffed bell peppers in a baking dish standing upright. If desired, place top back or cut reserve for a salad.

7. Place baking sheet in the oven and bake until the peppers are tender, about 30 – 35 minutes.

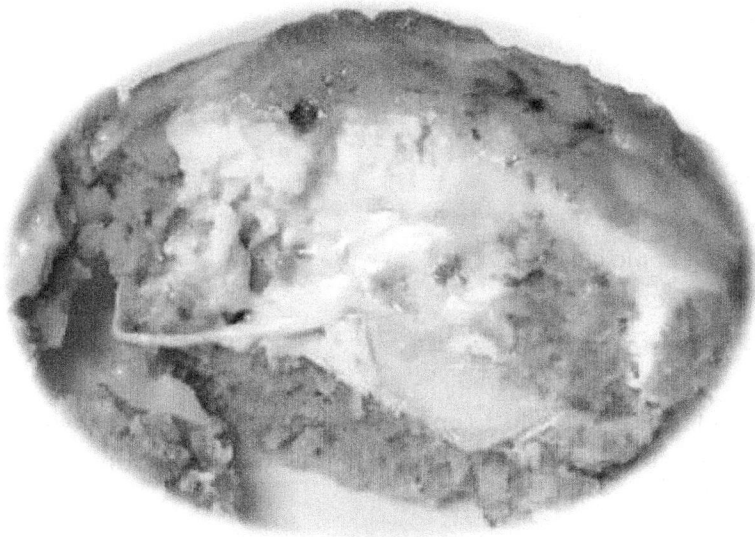

Maple Ground Beef Sausage

Prep time: 5 minutes

Cook time: 10 minutes

Servings: 12 servings per recipe

INGREDIENTS

1 tsp of water

2 tsp of maple syrup

1/4 tsp of ground all spice

1/4 tsp of mace or nutmeg

3/4 tsp of dried sage or 2 tbsp of fresh

1 tsp of white pepper

1/2 lbs of ground turkey

1 lbs of ground beef or pork

INSTRUCTIONS

1. In a large bowl, mix together the entire ingredients.

2. Place in the Refrigerator up to 4 hours or overnight.

3. Mold into patties, place in the skillet and cook over medium-high heat for about 10 minutes or until browned

Banana Coconut Muffins

Prep time: 5 minutes

Cook time: 25 minutes

Servings: 12

INGREDIENTS

½ tsp of baking soda

1 tsp of baking powder

½ tsp of salt

½ cup of coconut flour

2 tsp of vanilla extract

3 tbsp of maple syrup

4 ripe bananas, mashed

4 lightly beaten eggs

INSTRUCTIONS

1. Heat-up the oven to 325 F. Grease 2 muffin tins.

2. In a mixing bowl, combine together the vanilla extract, banana, eggs and maple syrup until well incorporated.

3. Stir the baking powder, coconut flour, baking soda and salt together in a mixing bowl.

4. Combine the dry ingredients into the wet ingredients and mix until fully combined. Let sit for 5 minutes.

5. Transfer batter into muffin tins.

6. Bake in the oven for 20- 25 minutes or until a knife inserted in the center comes out clean. Keep an eye on the muffins to ensure they do not get burnt.

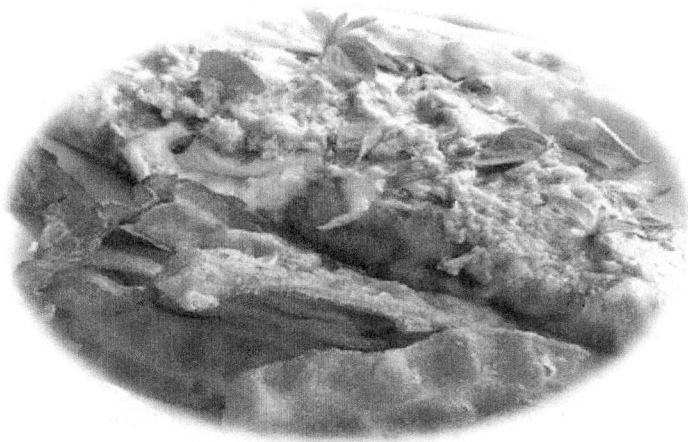

Mexican Brunch Eggs With Toasted bread

Servings: 8

INGREDIENTS

1/2 cup of onion, chopped

2 crushed cloves garlic

2 tbsp of margarine

1 1/2 cups of frozen corn, thawed

1 1/2 tsp of ground cumin

1/8 tsp of cayenne pepper

8 eggs, beaten

8 toasted bread slices

INSTRUCTIONS

1. Add the margarine in a large skillet and sauté onion and garlic until onion is soft.

2. Stir in cayenne, corn and cumin.

3. Add in eggs and cook, stirring periodically over low heat until eggs are set.

4. Place the toasted bread slices on a platter and spoon egg mixture over toast.

Cottage Cheese Pancakes

Prep Time: 5 minutes

Cook Time: 6 minutes

Servings: 6-8

INGREDIENTS

Butter, coconut oil, or ghee for frying

(Optional) 1/2 tsp of baking soda

Dash salt

1/2 cup of sweet rice flour or 1/4 cup of coconut flour

1 cup of cottage cheese

4 beaten eggs

INSTRUCTIONS

1. In a mixing bowl, mix the flour, cottage cheese, eggs and salt.

2. Place a skillet over medium heat, heat about half tablespoon of oil until it's hot.

3. Measure about 1/3 to 1/2 cup of the mixture into the pan. Cook about 3 or 4 minutes until golden brown underneath and it starts to bubble on top.

4. Flip and cook the other side for extra 1 to 2 minutes.

5. Serve with syrup and traditional butter, or sour cream, fresh fruit, honey or jam.

Morning Tostadas

Prep Time: 10 minutes

Cook Time: 10 minutes

Servings: 2

INGREDIENTS

Plain yogurt or sour cream

1/2 cup of low oxalate tomato (big beef is low oxalate tomato)

4 eggs

Pinch cayenne pepper

1 tbsp of fresh chopped fresh cilantro

1/4 cup of chopped red pepper

1/4 cup of chopped onion

2 oz of shredded mozzarella cheese of your choice

1 tbsp of olive oil, or butter

2 (7 or 8") white corn tortillas

INSTRUCTIONS

1. Heat olive oil or butter over medium low heat in a medium-sized skillet. Warm the corn tortillas in the skillet flip with tongs as soon as they are pliable.

2. Top each tortilla with 1 ounce shredded mozzarella cheese. Cover with a lid and let it cook for 1 minute. Set cooked tortillas aside on 2 plates.

3. Sweat the onions for 1-2 minutes in the skillet. Add chopped red pepper and cook for additional 1-2 minutes. Add in cayenne pepper and cilantro.

4. Gather the veggies towards a side in the pan add 4 eggs and cover with a lid. Cook for about 3 minute and flip eggs individually while yolk is still runny or slightly runny but button is set. Over easy or over medium eggs (instead, you can also scramble them).

5. Cook for additional 1 or 2 minutes or until yolk is set to desired "doneness."

6. Add half the veggies and two eggs on top each cheesy tortilla. Top with the tomatoes and dollop plain yogurt on top to garnish.

about 6.7 mg. oxalate per serving when using big beef tomatoes.

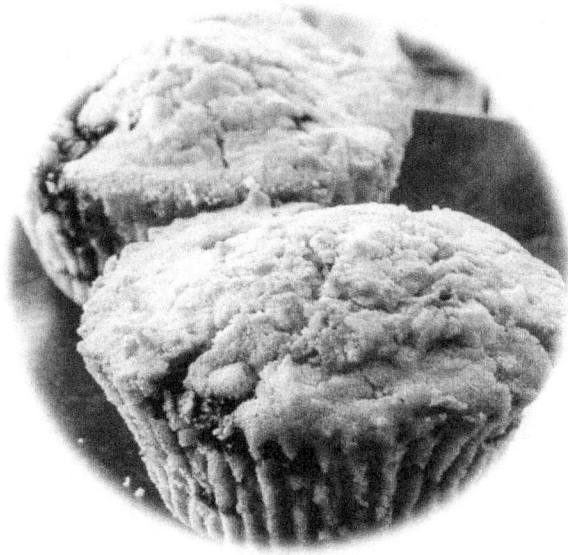

Mini Muffins

Prep Time: 8 minutes
Cook Time: 20 minutes
Servings: 12

INGREDIENTS

1/2 tsp of baking soda
1 tbsp of melted coconut oil
1/2 cup of ground pumpkin seeds
1/3 cup of applesauce
6-7 small (Neglet) dates, coarsely chopped

INSTRUCTIONS

1. Heat the oven to 375 degrees.

2. In the food processor, blend apple sauce and dates until well combined. (Pause a few times to unstick dates while blending.

3. Add the rest ingredients into the processor and blend until smooth.

4. Line mini muffin cups with cupcake or candy papers, fill muffin cups with the mixture until almost full. (It does not rise much).

5. Place in the oven and bake until a knife inserted to test the doneness comes out clean, about 20 minutes. They freeze great.

Vegetables Omelet Stuffing

Prep Time: 10 minutes

Cook Time: 8 minutes

Servings: 1

INGREDIENTS

1 Oz of shredded sharp cheddar cheese (low fat)

1 whole large egg

2 large egg whites

1/4 tsp of black pepper

2 tbsp of water

3 tbsp of chopped green onions

1/3 cup of chopped zucchini

1/4 cup of frozen whole-kernel corn, thawed

INSTRUCTIONS

1. Heat up your fry pan over high-medium heat. Smear cooking spray over the pan.

2. Add onions, zucchini, and corn, sauté vegetables until crisp-tender, about 4 minutes. Turn heat off.

3. Heat a nonstick skillet (10 inches) over high-medium heat.

4. In a bowl, combine pepper or extra spicy, water, egg and egg whites, whisk well.

5. Smear cooking spray over the pan and cook egg mixture, about 2 minutes in the pan until edges start to set. Lift the edges gently with a spatula, tilt pan around to allow uncooked side flow to the hot pan's surface.

6. Add vegetable to half of omelet, and then sprinkle sharp cheddar cheese over the vegetable mixture.

7. Use a spatula to loosen omelet edges and fold in half. Cook for extra 2 minutes to melt the cheese. Slide on a plate and enjoy.

Apple Nut Muffins

Prep Time: 10 minutes

Cook Time: 25 minutes

Servings: 12

INGREDIENTS

2 tbsp of oil

1/2 cup of molasses

1 beaten egg

2 cups of buttermilk or sour milk

1 orange juice

1/2 cup of chopped nuts

1/2 cup of raisins

1 cup of chopped apple

1/2 tsp of nutmeg

1 1/4 tsp of baking soda

1 1/2 cups of wheat bran

2 cups of whole wheat flour

INSTRUCTIONS

1. Heat up the oven to 350 F.

2. Combine together, flour, nutmeg bran, and baking soda with fork.

3. Stir in raisins, nuts or seeds, and apples.

4. Pour orange juice to fill a 2 cup measure and top with the buttermilk to complete the 2 cups.

5. Combine egg with orange juice buttermilk mixture, oil and molasses; stir well.

6. Stir wet mixture into dry mixture with a few swift strokes.

7. Fill mixture 2/3 full into greased muffin tins. Place in the oven and bake for 25 minutes.

VEGETABLES AND SALAD RECIPES

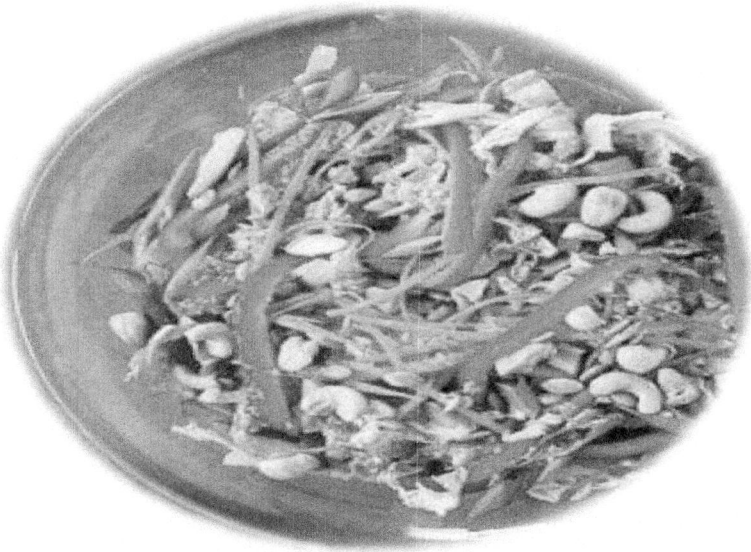

Cabbage Salad With Sesame Dressing

Prep Time: 10 minutes

Cook Time: 10 minutes

Servings: 6

INGREDIENTS

For the salad

(Optional) 1/4 cup of pepitas

1 cup of roughly chopped cilantro

4 green onions sliced thinly

1 deseeded and finely sliced red pepper

4 grated small carrots

4 cups of Napa cabbage finely shredded

2 tbsp of rice vinegar

2 tsp of sesame oil

3 tbsp of soy sauce or tamari organic

2 pkt of tempeh organic (450g total), cut into cubes

For the dressing

(Optional) squeeze lime juice

1/3 cup of water

1 tbsp of soy sauce or tamari organic.......check the oxalate contents

2 tbsp of honey raw

1 tbsp of sesame oil

3 tbsp of apple cider vinegar unpasteurized

1 tbsp of ginger finely diced (or 1 inch cube)

INSTRUCTIONS

1. Combine together the rice vinegar, sesame oil and soy sauce or tamari in a bowl. Place the tempeh in the mixture and let marinade for at least 10 minutes.

2. In a separate large bowl, combine the entire salad ingredients together. Add the seeds.

3. Heat a medium saucepan over medium heat. Add the marinated tempeh and fry until golden and crispy, about 10 minutes. Drizzle marinade on top tempeh as you cook.

4. Meanwhile, Combine the entire ingredients for the dressing together in a mason jar, close lid tightly and shake until well combined.

To serve, drizzle dressing over hot tempeh in individual bowl.

Coleslaw With Honey Mustard Dressing

Prep Time: 10 mins

Servings: 4-6

INGREDIENTS

Salad Mix

(Optional) ½ cup of red onions, thinly sliced

½ cup of green onions, sliced

8-10 thinly sliced radishes

½ head shredded or thinly sliced green cabbage

Dressing:

Salt and pepper to taste

2 tbsp of white wine vinegar

2 tsp of honey

2 tbsp of grainy Dijon mustard

½ cup of mayonnaise (Use high-quality)

INSTRUCTIONS

1. Combine the salad mix ingredients together in a bowl.

2. Whisk the entire ingredients for the dressing together in a bowl. Pour dressing over salad in a bowl and toss to coat. Season with salt and pepper.

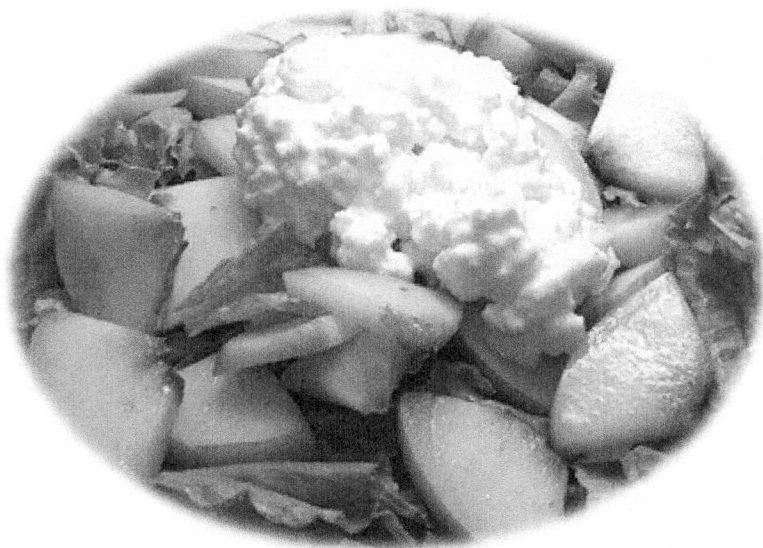

Watermelon Feta Salad

Prep Time: 15 minutes

Cook Time: 0 minutes

Servings: 6

INGREDIENTS

2 tbsp of extra virgin olive oil

1 tbsp of lime juice

1/8 tsp of white pepper

8 cups of cubed watermelon (about 1/2 of a medium watermelon)

1/4 cup of Kalamata olives

1/4 cup of red onions, sliced

1/4 packed cup of fresh mint, chopped

1/2 cup of feta cheese, cubed

INSTRUCTIONS

1. In a small bowl, whisk together the lime juice, olive oil and white pepper.

2. In a large serving bowl, combine the olives, cubed watermelon, mint and onions.

3. Spread lime/olive oil mixture over salad in the serving bowl and toss until well covered.

4. Add feta cubes into the bowl and carefully mix. Serve immediately.

Shallot Scallion Squash Salad

Time: 1 hour 30 minutes (make a day early)

Servings: 8-10

INGREDIENTS

(Optional) 1 medium organic Red Pepper, cut into ¼"x1 inch short strips or organic roasted red pepper

1 chopped Scallion, just the green part

½ cup of chopped Cilantro

½ finely diced medium Shallot, or 1 whole scallion (optional)

1 cup of red seedless grapes, cut in half, or ¼ cup of chopped cranberries or Raisins

1 (3 – 3½ pounds) of butternut squash seeded, peeled, and diced in 1" chunks

Dressing:

1/8 teaspoon of Cayenne Pepper or ¼ – ½ teaspoon of white pepper

¼ teaspoon of Cardamom

¼ teaspoon of ground Coriander

½ teaspoon of Mineral salt

2 tablespoons of Maple Syrup or 1½ tbsp of organic Sugar

¼ cup of Lime Juice

¼ cup of olive oil or more

INSTRUCTIONS

1. Boil squash in salted water for 5-7 minutes until soft but not mushy. Place cooked squash in the refrigerator to chill. This will keep the squash cubes more intact. To make the salad more colorful you can use both butternut and acorn squash (cooked separately)
2. In a bowl, mix together the entire dressing ingredients.
3. Add the squash cubes with other ingredients, then toss with the dressing to coat evenly.
4. Chill in the refrigerator about an hour. To served, garnish with grape halves or additional cilantro leaves or red pepper strips. Served chilled or at room temperature.

Mashed Avocado Egg Salad

Prep time: 10 minutes

Servings: 2

INGREDIENTS

1 cup of Arugula or Romaine (or any low oxalate green)

Salt to taste

5-6 hard-boiled eggs

1 tbsp of lemon juice

1/4 tsp of ground white pepper

1 tbsp of GF Dijon mustard or GF prepared yellow mustard

1 ripe avocado

INSTRUCTIONS

1. In a bowl, mash the avocado using a fork until mushy or you can make it a bit chunky.

2. Mix in the lemon juice, white pepper, mustard, and salt. Mash the eggs with a fork or chop them. Fold mashed/chopped eggs into the mixture until mixed well.

3. Serve on a bed of Arugula or Romaine with a few tablespoons yogurt. Best eaten right away or within few hours of preparing.

Lime Cilantro Slaw

Servings: 4

INGREDIENTS

1 tbsp of olive oil

1 1/2 tbsp of lime juice (about one lime)

1/4 cup of chopped cilantro

1 cup of chopped romaine lettuce

2 cups of chopped cabbage

INSTRUCTIONS

1. In a serving bowl, combine the lettuce, cilantro and cabbage.

2. Mix the olive oil and lime juice in a separate bowl.

3. Toss dressing with salad. Chill for few minutes before serving to blend flavors. Best eaten right away or within few hours of preparing.

Black Bean Corn Salad

Prep time: 15 minutes

Servings: 8

INGREDIENTS

1/4 tsp of cayenne pepper

2 tablespoons of lime juice (1 lime)

2 tbsp of extra-virgin olive oil

1/2 tsp of Celtic sea salt

3 minced cloves garlic,

1/4 cup of chopped fresh cilantro

3/4 cup of fresh corn, cut off the cob

2 cups of cooked black-eyed peas, rinsed

1 (about 1 cup) red pepper

INSTRUCTIONS

1. In a large salad bowl, combine black-eyed peas, cilantro, corn and red pepper; set aside.

2. Combine the olive oil, garlic and salt in a mortar or small bowl and smash everything together with a pestle until oil and salt is mixed with juice from garlic. If you don't have a pestle, you can also use the back of a spoon.

3. Mix together the cayenne pepper and lime juice until well mix.

4. Drizzle the dressing on top black-eyed peas mixture and gently toss to coat.

If desired, serve salad with corn tortillas, sliced avocado and Lime Cilantro Slaw.

Brussel Sprouts With Bacon

Prep time: 10 minutes

Cook time: 30 minutes

INGREDIENTS

1 tbsp of thyme

2 minced cloves garlic

1/2 cup of chicken broth or pork broth, or water

1/2 tsp of celtic sea salt

1 1/2 lbs of Brussels sprouts, cut in quarters and ends trimmed or cauliflower for a lower version

1/2 lbs of diced bacon

INSTRUCTIONS

1. Add the bacon in a skillet and brown bacon until crispy.

2. Add Brussels sprouts in a large saucepan and boil for about 10 minutes. Drain water from the Brussels sprouts and mix with the cooked bacon, along with the juice from cooking with the rest ingredients. Mix until finely coated.

3. Transfer coated mixture into a ceramic or glass baking dish.

4. Place baking dish in the oven and bake for about 30 minutes at 350 degrees.

Recipe Note: For lower oxalate content, replace brussel sprouts with cauliflower or use 1/2 of both. Brussels sprouts are lower in oxalate content when boiled compare to steaming. Boiling 1/2 cup of Brussels sprout gives you about 8.5 mg while steaming gives you 12.7 mg.

Pear And wine vinegar Arugula Salad

Servings: 6

INGREDIENTS

1 minced shallot

1 sliced pear

6 cups of arugula (Rinse and trimmed stems off)

3 tablespoon of red wine vinegar

Cracked black pepper

1 teaspoon of Dijon mustard

2/3 cup of extra virgin olive oil

INSTRUCTIONS

1. Combine Dijon mustard, black pepper, red wine vinegar and shallot in blender. Fold in the olive oil to emulsify.

2. Combine together arugula and pear and toss to coat with the dressing.

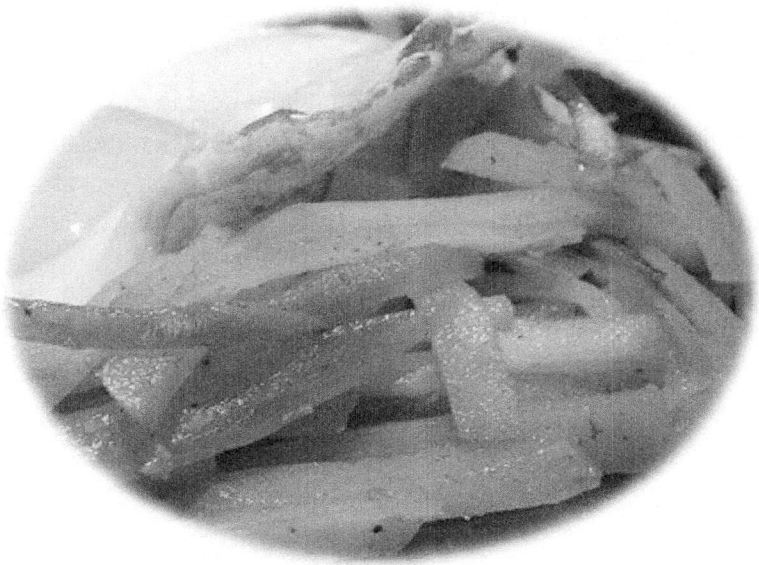

Crispy Kohlrabi

Prep time: 15 minutes

Cook time: 35-40 minutes

Servings: 6

INGREDIENTS

(Optional) 1/2 tsp of thyme

1/2 tsp of white pepper

1/4 tsp of salt or more to taste

1 minced clove garlic

 2 tbsp of olive oil

3 cups of kohlrabi

INSTRUCTIONS

1. Remove the tough skin off kohlrabi to access the inside juicy flesh. Cut the kohlrabi into half inch pieces. Set aside in a bowl.

2. In a bowl, add the garlic, olive oil, thyme, salt and pepper and mix well.

3. Spread the oil mixture over kohlrabi slices in the bowl and toss until all pieces are coated.

4. You either braise the kohlrabi over medium heat in a skillet until the kohlrabi is fork tender or Roast for about 35-40 minutes at 400 degrees in a baking sheet, stirring each 6-8 minutes interval after 20 minutes until fork tender.

MAIN DISH

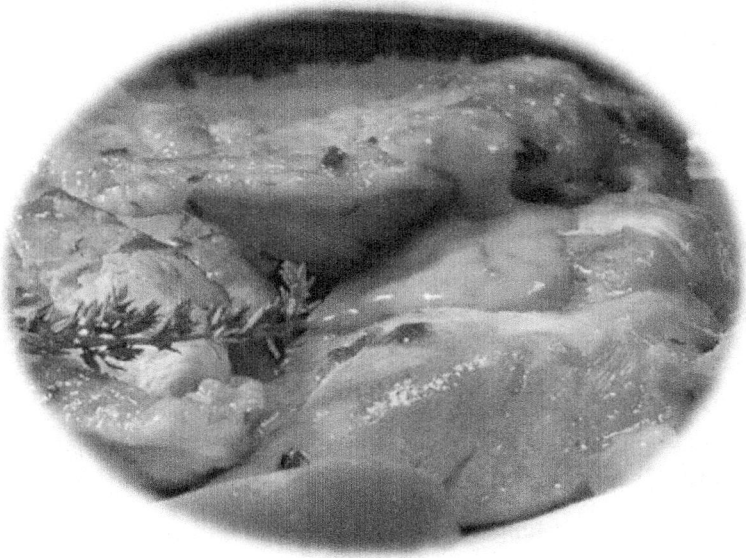

Spicy Steamed Fish

Prep Time: 7 minutes

Cook Time: 7 minutes

Servings: 4

INGREDIENTS

1 cup of hot water

1 tablespoon of lime juice

1 tablespoon of Ketchup

1 large sprig thyme

1 teaspoon of hot pepper sauce

¼-1/2 teaspoon of white pepper

1/2 cup sliced onion

3/4 (175 ml) cup of red and green peppers, sliced

1/2 cup of olive oil, (125 ml)

4 (100 g per fillet) fillets of tilapia

INSTRUCTIONS

1. Sautee onion and bell peppers in olive oil in a fry pan over medium heat.

2. Add ketchup, thyme, hot pepper sauce, white pepper, half cup hot water and lime juice, Stir.

3. Add the fillets of tilapia in pan and pour in half cup of the hot water, spoon sauce and vegetables over fish.

4. Place the lid and cook for 5 minutes. Flip fish, cover and cook for extra 5 minutes.

Easy Fajitas Meal

Prep time: 10 minutes

Cook time: 15-20 minutes

Servings: 4 (2 fajitas each).

INGREDIENTS

Cilantro to taste

Sour cream to taste

8 corn tortillas

2 sliced bell peppers

1 sliced onion

1 lbs. of meat, tofu, shrimp bite sizes

Dash cayenne pepper

1 tsp of cumin

1 lemon or orange zest and juice

1 lime zest and juice

1 tbsp of olive oil

INSTRUCTIONS

1. In a small bowl, combine together cumin, citrus juice and zest, oil, and cayenne pepper.

2. Pour the marinade in a shallow dish or bag, add the vegetables and meat and marinate overnight.

3. Cook the marinated vegetables and meat over medium heat in a large skillet for about 15-20 minutes or until onions are soft and starting to caramelize and the meat is cooked.

4. Spoon into tortillas and serve with cilantro and sour cream over the top.

Garbanzo Bean Parsley Salad

Prep Time: 15 minutes

Servings: 6

INGREDIENTS

1/2 cup of chopped parsley

10 black olives

3 minced garlic cloves

1/2 teaspoon of black pepper

1/2 teaspoon of sea salt

1 teaspoon of ground cumin

1/4 cup of extra virgin olive oil

1/4 cup of freshly squeezed lime juice

1 cup of cherry or grape tomatoes

1 cup of diced sweet yellow onion

1 red bell pepper, chopped

1 green bell pepper, chopped

2 (15 ounce) cans of garbanzo beans, drained

INSTRUCTIONS

1. In a non-metallic large mixing bowl, combine together the green peppers and red peppers, cherry, garbanzo beans, onion, chopped parsley and olives.

2. Pulse the olive oil, cumin, minced garlic, lime juice, salt and pepper in a blender until desired consistency is achieved.

3. Spread dressing over salad. Cover and chill in the refrigerator for 60 to 120 minutes.

Friendly Beef Stew

Prep Time: 60 minutes

Cook Time: 1 hour 30 minutes

Servings: 8

INGREDIENTS

1/2 tsp of Celtic sea salt

2 cups of sliced mushrooms

2 cups of yellow onions, chopped

4-6 ounces diced bacon

1/2 tsp of freshly ground black pepper

1 tsp of thyme

1 bay leaf

6 – 8 large cloves garlic

2 tbsp of olive oil

2 cups of dry, red wine

2 pounds boneless beef stew meat, cubed

INSTRUCTIONS

1. Combine the red wine, black pepper, olive oil, cloves garlic, bay leaf and thyme in a bowl. Add beef stew meat, cover and refrigerate for 1 to 24 hours, turning periodically. Drain beef and reserve liquid.

2. Cook the bacon over medium heat in a large Dutch oven until bacon is brown. Remove bacon and set aside.

3. Add cooked beef to the juice that came from cooking the bacon and cook until starting to brown.

4. Add the chopped onions and sliced mushrooms and cook until onions are translucent and beef is browned.

5. Add the marinade, bacon and season with salt, bring to a boil. Turn heat down and cook covered for about 60 to 90 minutes or until the meat is tender. Season with more salt if needed and cook until liquid is reduced to desired consistency.

6. Serve over the top of mashed cauliflower or with cooked greens or butternut squash.

Zucchini Ground Turkey Pizza Casserole

Prep Time: 10 minutes
Cook Time:20 minutes
Servings: 8

INGREDIENTS

1 clove garlic
1/2 cup Parmesan cheese grated
1 can of del monte diced tomatoes no salt
1/2 cup of Free fat shredded cheese
16 ounces of ground turkey 93% fat free
1/2 cup of Egg Beaters
2 cups of Zucchini squash, shredded

INSTRUCTIONS

1. Heat-up the oven to 400 F. Grease a 9 x 11 baking dish with nonstick spray.
2. Cook the sausage in a non-stick pan over a medium heat, about 15 to 20 minutes; drain and rinse.
3. Shred the zucchini by hand or add to a food processor. Set aside on a paper towel to drain. Drain water out of the tomatoes.
4. Mix together ground turkey, egg Beaters, Zucchini squash, drained tomatoes, free fat shredded cheese and garlic.
5. Pour the mixture onto the prepared baking dish. Sprinkle top of mixture with Parmesan cheese.
6. Place dish in the oven and bake for approximate 20 minutes or until no more moisture on top. The cooking time will depend on how well you blot the zucchini.

Low Oxalate Souffle

Prep Time: 10 minutes

Total Time: 50 minutes

Servings: 10

INGREDIENTS

1 tsp of black pepper

9 tbsp of margarine

9 tbsp of white flour (whole wheat flour can be substituted)

9 medium eggs, whites separated from yolks

2 cups of fresh turkey breast meat, cut into cubes

1 tsp of salt

INSTRUCTIONS

1. Heat up the oven to 350 F. Greased a 4-6 quart baking dish.

2. Heat margarine over medium heat in a 2 quart saucepan, once melted add in flour, stirring frequently until you have a creamy mixture. Remove from heat.

3. Gently stir in egg yolks, add the whites and keep stirring.

4. Add in turkey cubes and mix thoroughly until well mixed.

5. Transfer mixture into the baking dish.

6. Bake without covering for 45 minutes or until lightly browned on top and a toothpick used as a tested dipped in the center comes out clean.

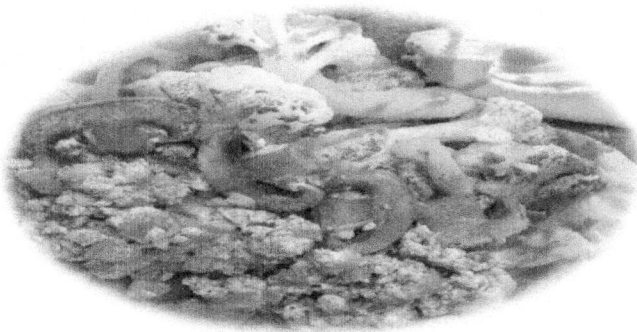

Broccoli Onion Beef

Prep Time: 10 minutes

Cook Time: 6 minutes

Servings: 6

INGREDIENTS

1/2 tsp of white pepper

(Optional) 1/8 tsp of cayenne pepper

1 tbsp of sesame oil

1/4 cup of Coconut Aminos

3 – 4 cups of broccoli florets or 12 – 16 oz. bag, frozen

3/4 cup of coarsely chopped onion

1.5 pounds of flank steak, cut against the grain

1 tbsp of raw ginger, minced

5 minced cloves garlic

2 tbsp of olive oil

Salt to taste

INSTRUCTIONS

1. Cook the garlic and ginger in hot oil over medium heat in a large skillet or wok, stirring constantly for 1 minute.

2. Add flank steak and stir-fry about 2-3 minutes until browned. Add the chopped onions and broccoli florets and stir-fry for about 1-2 minutes.

3. Add sesame oil, coconut aminos, 1 or 2 pinches of white pepper and cayenne pepper, stirring continuously for 1-3 more minutes until onions and broccoli are soft. Taste and adjust seasonings, if needed.

Lemon Parmesan Zoodles

Prep Time: 10 minutes

Cook Time: 5 minutes

Servings: 4

INGREDIENTS

1/4 cup of shredded parmesan cheese

4 cloves garlic, finely minced

1/4 cup of low-sodium vegetable stock

1 lemon juice

2 tbsp of unsalted butter, melted

2-3 large zucchini

Salt and white pepper

INSTRUCTIONS

1. Slice the zucchini into thin noodles using a spiralizer.

2. Heat the butter in a large sauté pan over medium-low heat, add garlic and cook until garlic is fragrant.

3. Add the vegetable stock, lemon juice, salt, and white pepper. Simmer over medium heat for 2 minutes or until liquid has reduced.

4. Add zucchini slices and toss to coat with the sauce. Sprinkle with extra white pepper and parmesan cheese if desired. Serve with shrimp or chicken.

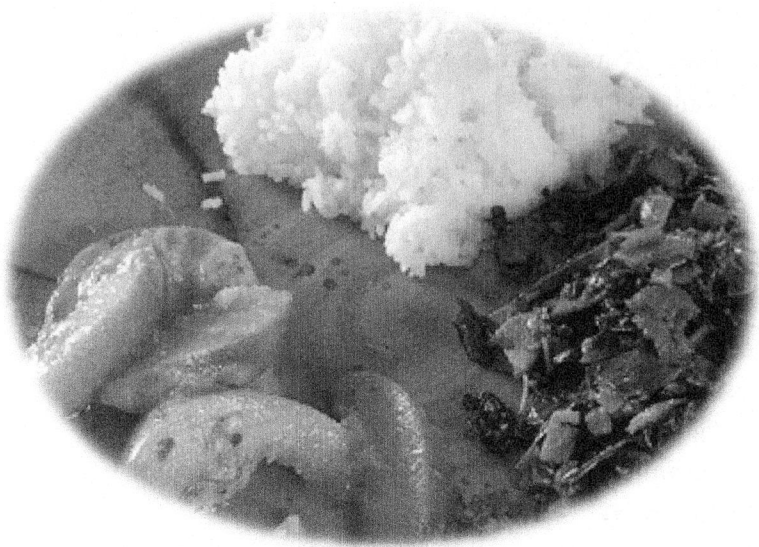

Chicken Ginger Mushrooms Stir-fry

Prep Time: 15 minutes

Cook Time: 15 minutes

Servings: 4

INGREDIENTS

Stir-fry Mix

1 package of rice noodles

2 tbsp of vegetable oil

1 handful of enoki mushrooms

1/2 cup of slant cut green onions

3 cups of cauliflower florets

2 cups of peeled carrots (moderate when cook but high when raw)

4 cups of sliced cremini mushrooms

4 cups of sliced purple cabbage

1 pounds of cooked chicken

Stir-fry Sauce

1 tbsp of vegetable oil

(Optional) 1 tsp of favorite hot sauce

1 cup of chicken stock

1/4 cup of rice wine vinegar

1/4 cup of honey

1/4 tsp of grated ginger

4 minced garlic cloves

INSTRUCTIONS

Stir-fry Sauce

1. In a small pot, heat the oil with the garlic on low-medium heat until garlic is brown and sticky but not black.

2. Pour in honey and allow for a moment to bubble. Add rice wine vinegar and cover with a lid so you won't get burnt by the bubbling.

3. Add the chicken stock and cook until liquid is reduced by half. Add salt and pepper to taste along with your desired hot sauce.

Stir-fry Mix

4. Cook the noodles as instructed in package directions. Drain, and set aside to cool.

5. Pour the oil in a large wok and heat over medium heat. Add the vegetables and stir-fry, starting with the hardest or longest to cook. Make sure the pan is not too stuff with vegetables or you can cook in batches if your wok is not large enough.

6. Once vegetables are tender and caramelized, add noodles with chicken. Stir in the sauce until well mixed. Do not cook to reduce sauce again so that it won't get too salty.

Broccoli With Cranberries

Prep Time: 5 minutes

Cook Time: 5 minutes

Servings: 4

INGREDIENTS

1/2 cup of sweetened dried cranberries

4 cups of broccoli florets

3 minced cloves garlic

2 tsp of olive oil

INSTRUCTIONS

1. Heat the oil over medium heat in a large skillet and sauté the garlic in hot oil for about 1 minute. Add broccoli florets and cranberries and return to sauté for about 3 minutes, until broccoli is tender and crispy. Season with salt and pepper to taste.

Lemon Dilled Fish

Prep time: 5 mins

Cook time: 17-20 mins

Servings: 6

INGREDIENTS

4 tsp of lemon juice

Dash of pepper

1/2 tsp of dill weed

1/4 tsp of mustard powder

1 tsp of instant onion, (freeze dried) minced

1 1/2 lbs or fresh, firm white fish

INSTRUCTIONS

1. Heat up the oven to 475 F.

2. Wash the fish well and pat dry.

3. Place fish in a baking dish.

4. Combine 2 tablespoons of water, dill weed, mustard pepper and onion, add in lemon juice and spread evenly on top of the fish.
5. Place in the oven and bake uncovered for 17-20 minutes.

Shrimp Linguine

Servings: 2 servings per recipe

High Protein, Low Phosphorus, Low Potassium,

INGREDIENTS

¼ cup of chopped cilantro

2 cups of cooked linguine

¼ cup of 10% table cream

¼ cup of prepared salsa (hot, med or mild)

1 pepperoncini or pickled jalapeno pepper

1 small minced clove garlic

1 Tablespoon of canola oil

12 large shrimp, cut into bit-sized pieces

INSTRUCTIONS

1. Cook pasta the way instructed in the package.
2. While the pasta is cooking, in a medium-sized sauté pan, sauté shrimp in oil over medium-high heat.
3. When shrimp color is turning orange/pink, add salsa, pepperoncini and garlic, then turn to low heat. Cook until shrimps are totally cooked.
4. Once the pasta is ready, remove from heat and mix the table cream and pasta into the shrimp mixture. Stir well to coat. Sprinkle with fresh cilantro and serve.

Salmon Cucumber Salad

Prep Time: 10 minutes

Cook Time: 15 to 20 minutes

Servings: 4

INGREDIENTS

½ cup of salmon, low sodium, drained

1 cooked egg, chopped

½ cup of celery, chopped

½ teaspoon of celery seed

1 teaspoon of horseradish

½ cup of sliced cucumber

1 tablespoon of finely chopped onion

¼ teaspoon of pepper

¼ cup of French dressing

½ cup of rice, uncooked

INSTRUCTIONS

1. Pour two cups of water and rice in a saucepan. Cover with the lid and bring to a boil. Reduce heat to low and simmer, about 15 to 20 minutes until rice is cooked.

2. Transfer rice to a bowl, cover and let sit for 15 minutes.

3. Add the French dressing and allow cooling and then add the rest ingredients.

Allow to chill in the refrigerator for up to an hour.

Rice And Peas

Prep Time: 10 minutes

Cook Time: 60 minutes

Servings: 4 main dish or 8 side dish servings

INGREDIENTS

1/4 teaspoon sea salt or more to taste

2-4 crushed cloves garlic

1 tsp of dried thyme

(Optional) 1 habanero pepper

2 cups of long grain white rice (not instant!)

1 cup of water

1 (13.5 ounces) can of unsweetened coconut Milk

2 cups of cooked black-eyed peas or pigeon peas or kidney beans

INSTRUCTIONS

1. Add the entire ingredients along with liquid from the cooked beans, (if any) into a saucepan. (The liquid should measure up to 3/4 cup liquid, add water if necessary).

2. Bring mixture to a boil, reduce heat and simmer on low for about 30 minutes or until rice is tender and most of the liquid has evaporate. Discard the habanero pepper and serve.

Mushroom Chicken in Slow Cooker

Prep Time: 5 minutes

Cook Time: 8 minutes

Servings: 6

INGREDIENTS

4 cups of low-sodium organic chicken broth

1 white onion, chopped into small pieces

1 minced clove of garlic

2 large chicken breasts

1 cup of sliced mushrooms

1/2 cup of corn

1/2 cup of peas

Salt and white pepper to taste

INSTRUCTIONS

1. Add the onion, garlic, chicken breasts, corn, mushroom, peas, and pepper and salt in a 5-quart slow cooker. Cook on low for 6 hours or 2 hours on high.

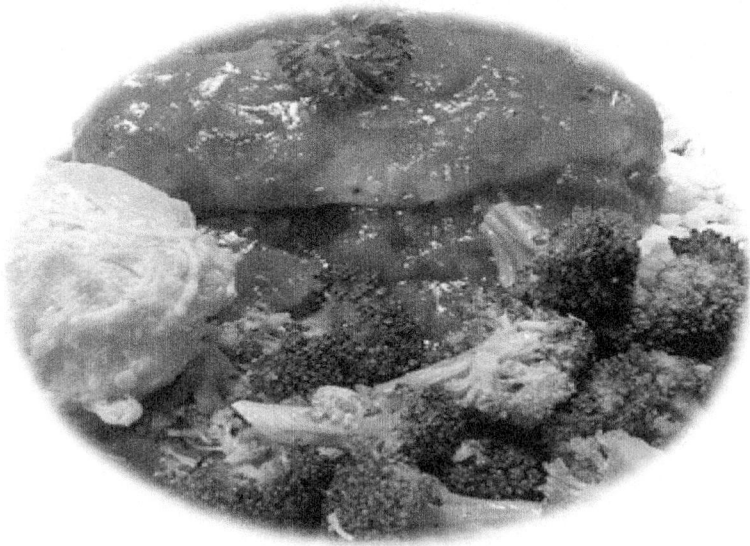

Rice With Spiced Mung Beans

Prep Time: 9 hours
Total Time: 45 minutes
Servings: 6-8

INGREDIENTS

1 cup of mung beans (medium oxalate food with 7.9 mg, soaked overnight)
3 tbsp of butter (or cooking oil of your choice)
1 ½ tsp of grated ginger
1 bay leaf
2 cups of long grain rice
½-1 tsp of nutmeg
1/4 – 1/2 teaspoon cardamom (optional)
¼ teaspoon cayenne pepper
1 teaspoon salt
¼ cup onion, chopped
1 – 2 hard-boiled eggs

INSTRUCTIONS

1. Soak the beans in water for at least 8 hours or overnight. OR bring to a boil in a large pot filled with about 4 cups water. Remove from heat and allow sit for 60 minutes. Drain beans and rinse.
2. Heat the butter over medium heat in a Dutch oven or large saucepan. Add bay leaf and ginger and sauté for 1 minute.
3. Add the soaked and drained beans, rice, cardamom, cinnamon and pepper, and cook stirring occasionally for 12 – 15 minutes. Add about 6 cups of water, season with salt and bring mixture to a boil.
4. Cover pot with a lid and simmer for about 30 minutes on low heat or until the beans and rice are tender.
5. While the beans and rice is cooking, fry the onion in a little oil in a separate skillet. Serve meal in serving dish and garnish with slices of hard-boiled egg fried and onions.

Note: You may substitute mung beans for lentils. You do not need to be pre-soaked the lentils.

Grilled Salmon With Pear

Prep Time: 20 minutes

Cook Time: 10 minutes

Servings: 4

INGREDIENTS

3/4 cup of olive oil

1/4 cup of balsamic vinegar

1 clove garlic

2 tbsp of lemon juice

2 tbsp of honey

1/2 tsp of white pepper

4 (4 oz each) fresh salmon fillets

4 cup of iceberg lettuce

2 ripe California Bartlett pears, cut in half and core

INSTRUCTIONS

1. In a small bowl, combine together the lemon juice, olive oil, balsamic vinegar, garlic, honey and pepper. Set aside.

2. Brush the salmon fillets with olive oil then sprinkle with white pepper.

3. Prepare your grill by brushing the grate with olive oil.

4. Place the salmon fillets and grill until lightly browned, about 3 to 4 minutes. Carefully turn the salmon over and grill for additional 3 to 5 minutes.

5. Place the pear halves on a pre-heated grill facing down, and grill for 3 to 5 minutes.

6. Arrange four serving bowls and divide Iceberg lettuce amongst each bowls.

7. Serve the grilled salmon over the bed of lettuce along with each pear half. Drizzle top with balsamic/lemon mix.

Bananas Cherries Balls

Servings: 12 balls

INGREDIENTS

1 egg white

1/4 teaspoon of cayenne pepper

1/4 teaspoon of ground cinnamon

1/2 teaspoon of real vanilla extract

3/4 cup of canned cherries, chopped

1/2 cup of raisins, sultana

4 rice cakes, whole wheat or white

1 cup of banana chips

4 tbsp of room temperature butter, cut into small cubes

4 peeled bananas cut lengthwise in half

INSTRUCTIONS

1. Preheat oven broiler. Place banana halves baking tray, sprinkle with cinnamon and cayenne. Broil until bananas are fully caramelized, about 5-7 minutes. Let sit for few minutes.

2. Heat the oven to 350 F. In a food processor, blend 2 tablespoons of the cubed butter with the bananas until smooth. Set aside.

3. In the blender, pulse the banana chips until you achieve a desired consistency. Add rice cakes into the blender and blend to have chunky texture.

4. Transfer onto the baking tray and bake about 10 minutes or until crispy.

5. Mix the rice cake mixture and banana mixture together along with the remaining ingredients until well incorporate.

6. Mold mixture into about 2 ounces balls. Place pan in the oven and bake for 10 to 13 minutes. Let cool before serving.

Chicken Hot Sauce Enchiladas

Prep Time: 5 minutes

Cook Time: 30 minutes

Servings: 10

INGREDIENTS

½ cup of hot sauce

⅓ to ½ cup of hot sauce for the top

10 wraps (coconut Paleo Wraps work well)

1 lbs of chopped cooked chicken, or shredded

8 oz of grated cheese, divided

2 teaspoons of black cumin seeds (nigella sativa optional)

1 whole roasted red pepper, diced

½ cup of cooked squash (or more)

½ cup of cooked lentils

1 medium onion, diced into ¼ inch

2 tablespoons of ghee

Salt to taste

INSTRUCTIONS

1. Heat the oven to 350 degrees F°. Heat the ghee in the saucepan over medium heat and sauté the onions until soft.

2. In a bowl, mix together the entire ingredients with the exception of the wraps, (4 ounces) second half of cheese and the final hot sauce in the saucepan used to sauté the onions.

3. Roll half cup of the stuffing into each wraps, roll wraps firmly to allow stuffing go in way to the end (if not done properly, it will burn)

4. Place stuffs wraps in a 9×13 baking dish and line them up closely.

5. Spread top of wraps with the remaining hot sauce and sprinkle with reserved cheese.

6. Place in the oven and bake about 15-20 minutes or until cheese melts. Keep a close eye to avoid burning the wraps

SOUP RECIPES

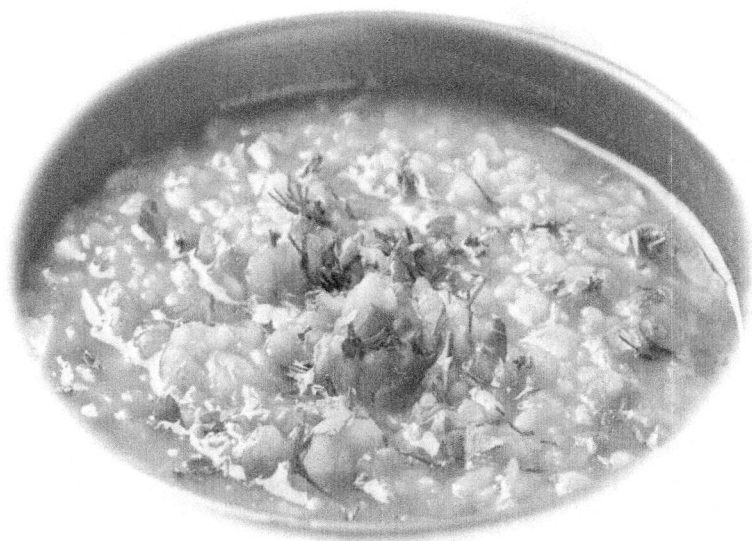

My Chili Soup

Prep Time: 5 minutes

Cook Time: 14 minutes

Servings: 12

INGREDIENTS

1 ½ cup of pumpkin puree

16 ounces package of frozen black-eyed peas

1 tsp of dried basil

2 cup of homemade beef broth or low sodium beef broth

½ cup of lentils

½ tsp of cayenne pepper

1 tbsp of chili powder

3 minced garlic cloves

1 small red bell pepper

1 red onion, chopped

1 pounds of ground turkey

1 tbsp of coconut oil

INSTRUCTIONS

1. Add coconut oil in a large saucepan over medium-high heat, once hot, add the onion, ground turkey, red bell pepper, garlic, chilli pepper, cayenne pepper and lentils; cook stirring frequently, until meat crumbles and is no more pink.

2. Add the rest ingredients into the saucepan and bring mixture to a boil.

3. Turn heat down and simmer for 30 minutes over medium, stirring occasionally until sauce has thickened. Serve with desired toppings in soup bowls.

Heart Warming Pea Soup

Prep Time: 5 minutes

Total Time: 18 minutes

Servings: 6

INGREDIENTS

1 onion, chopped

2 cups of homemade chicken broth

1 cup of cooked chicken, chopped

2 (16 ounces) packages of frozen green peas

2 (16 ounces) packages of frozen cauliflower

1 quart of water

Salt to taste

INSTRUCTIONS

1. Boil the peas in a sauce pan for 2-3 minutes until soft. Drain.

2. Boil the cauliflower and onions in 1 quart water until soft, reserve cooking liquid.

3. Puree the onion, cauliflower, chicken broth and cooking liquid until smooth.

4. Add the cooked chicken, and cooked peas and cauliflower stock to the sauce pan, season with salt to taste. Simmer for 10-15 minutes on low heat.

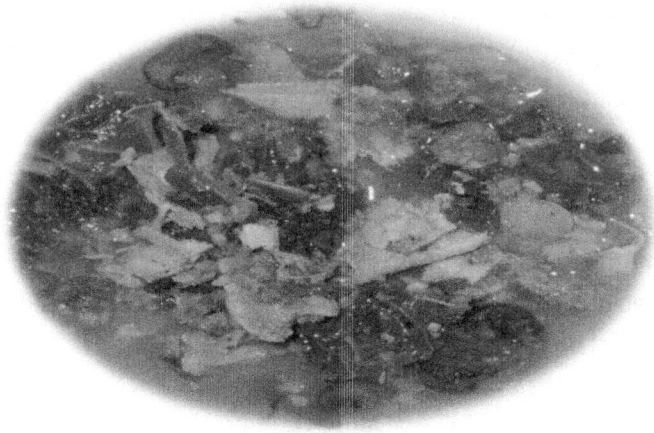

Quick Salmon Soup

Prep Time: 5 minutes

Cook Time: 5 minutes

Servings: 4

INGREDIENTS

Hot pepper sauce

¼ – ½ tsp of salt, to taste

1/8 tsp of white pepper

1¼ cups of chicken bone broth or fish stock plus 1 13.5 ounces can of coconut milk

1 – 2 tsp of fresh lemon juice

4 – 6 tablespoons of organic grass-fed butter or ghee

14 3/4 oz of red or pink wild-caught salmon, drain and reserve the liquid

INSTRUCTIONS

1. Melt the butter or ghee in a heavy skillet over low- medium heat.

2. Debone the salmon and gently crush bones using back of a spoon.

3. Add salmon flesh along with crushed bones to the butter; break salmon into small pieces.

4. Add drained fish liquid and chicken bone broth or fish stock with milk and stir repeatedly as it heat until hot.(Do not boil).Turn heat off; Season with salt, fresh lemon juice and pepper. Garnish with hot bacon or finely chopped paprika or chives, if desired.

Note: 3 cups of fresh unprocessed whole-fat milk can be substituted for the chicken bone broth or fish stock and coconut milk.

Seafood Turkey Fiesta

Prep time: 15 minutes

Cook time: 32 minutes

Servings: 12, one cup servings

INGREDIENTS

3 cups of chopped eggplant

6 oz of canned crab, drained

1/2 lbs of cooked shrimp

2 quarts of low sodium chicken broth

1 tbsp of salt-free Cajun seasoning

1/2 cup of flour

1/2 cup of canola oil

8 oz of sliced lean smoked turkey sausage

2 skinless chicken breasts, chopped

1 chopped red bell pepper

1 chopped yellow onion

3 chopped celery stalks

1 tbsp of canola oil

INSTRUCTIONS

1. In a large pot, heat 1 tablespoon of canola oil over medium- high heat.

2. Add onion, sausage, chicken, bell pepper and celery, cook for 10 minutes. Transfer mixture into a bowl and set aside.

3. Reduce to medium-low heat and add half cup of canola oil, then stir in flour to make a roux.

4. Mix in the Cajun seasoning, cook for 1 or more minutes, then stir in chicken broth, (Very slowly) stirring frequently to make sure no lumps forms.

5. Increase to high-medium- heat and cook until it starts to thicken slightly, about 10 minutes.

6. Lower to medium-low heat and add crab, okra and shrimp, add the chicken mixture earlier set aside and cook for 10 minutes or until cooked through.

Alfredo Sauce Soup

Servings: 8

INGREDIENTS

2 tbsp of chopped basil

1 tbsp of lemon juice

1/4 tsp of ground nutmeg

1/3 cup plus two tbsp of shredded parmesan cheese, divided

4 oz of cream cheese

2 cups of milk

1 minced garlic clove

3 tbsp of all-purpose flour

1/4 cup of olive oil

INSTRUCTIONS

1. Heat oil over medium heat in a large pan. Make a paste by adding flour and then whisk and add minced garlic.

2. Whisk milk slowly, whisking frequently so no lumps form. Let mixture heat up and thicken, then add in your cream cheese and whisk to combine. Turn off the heat.

3. Add lemon juice, nutmeg and 1/3 cup parmesan cheese. Stir well to combine.

4. Serve over steamed vegetables, chicken, pasta etc.

5. Garnish with the remaining parmesan cheese and chopped basil.

Black-eyed Peas White Chicken Chili

Prep Time: 10 minutes

Cook Time: 1 hour 15 minutes

Servings: 8

INGREDIENTS

(Optional) 4 ounces shredded cheese for garnish

(Optional) 1/4 cup of chopped fresh cilantro

1-2 cups of cooked black-eyed peas

1 tbsp of juice of a half lime

1/2 tsp of ground oregano (1 tsp if using fresh)

(Optional) 1/8 – 1/4 tsp of ground cayenne pepper

2 – 4 cups of homemade chicken broth (or Swansons 100% Natural)

1 (4 ounces) can of chopped green chiles (or use 2-3 fresh)

4-6 crushed cloves garlic

1 cup of chopped onion

1 tbsp of olive oil

1 1/2 lbs of boneless chicken breasts or thighs, cut into bite-sized pieces

INSTRUCTIONS

1. Heat olive oil in a large soup pot over medium heat. Cook the chicken in hot oil, stirring periodically for about 5-8 until the chicken starts to brown.

2. Add in the chopped onions, green chiles and garlic and cook for additional 3-5 minutes until chicken is lightly browned and onions are soft and translucent.

3. Add the oregano, cayenne pepper, lime juice, chicken broth and cooked black-eyed peas (You can add the liquid from cooking if you like).

4. Let soup simmer on medium low heat for about 45 minutes to 1 hour or until liquid has reduced about 1/5 to 1/4. Serve in bowls and top with cheese and cilantro if desired.

Note: if you wish to reduce the oxalate content of this soup, increase the cayenne to 1/2 tsp. and leave out the green chilies.

Chicken With Mushrooms Soup

Prep time: 15 minutes

Cook time: 20-25 minutes

Servings: 6

INGREDIENTS

1 chopped lemon grass stalk

1/2 sliced yellow onion

1 sliced red bell pepper

10 white button mushrooms, quartered

2 tbsp of lime juice

1 inch sliced ginger

1 tsp of chili sauce or chili flakes

1 lbs of chicken breast or shrimp, cut into bite size pieces

1 tbsp of brown or white sugar

1/2 tbsp of fish sauce

4 cups of low sodium broth or Simple Chicken Broth

1 can of lite coconut milk

INSTRUCTIONS

1. Spray a nonstick cooking spray on a large pot, add shrimp or chicken and cook over medium heat until evenly browned.

2. Add ginger, lemongrass, chili sauce, sugar, fish sauce, and broth. Bring to a boil.

3. Reduce to low-medium heat and simmer about 10 to 15 minutes.

4. Add onion, bell pepper, mushrooms and coconut milk and simmer for 5 more minutes.

5. Mix in lime juice just before serving.

Corn Onion Fennel Soup

Prep time: 12 minutes

Cook time: 30-35 minutes

Servings: 12

INGREDIENTS

2 liters of cold water

Tarragon to taste

Black pepper to taste

2 cups of chopped fennel

6 cloves garlic

1 chopped celery stalk

2 chopped onions or leeks

2 pounds of frozen corn

2 tablespoon of vegetable oil

Shrimp shells

INSTRUCTIONS

1. Add oil in a sauce pan and sauté shrimp shells until color turns pink.

2. Add onion, garlic, corn, celery and fennel and sauté until onions are tender and translucent and flavored.

3. Add in water and bring to a boil. Simmer for about 30 minutes.

4. Transfer soup to a blender (be careful of the hot liquid) and blend.

5. Strain soup to remove any excess fibers.

6. Adjust seasonings with tarragon and ground black pepper.

SIDE DISH AND SNACKS RECIPES

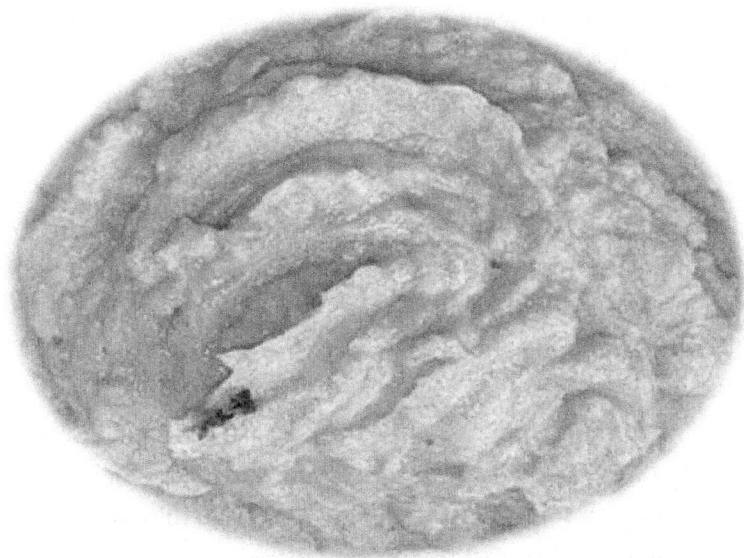

Cauliflower Pumpkin Hummus

Prep Time: 20 minutes

Cook Time: 30 minutes

Servings: 8 -10

INGREDIENTS

½ Cup of coarsely chopped cilantro leaves (tightly packed)

1/8 tsp of cayenne pepper or a rounded ¼ tsp of white pepper

1 tsp of mineral salt (if seeds are unsalted)

3 tbsp of lemon juice

3 tbsp of olive oil

(Optional) 2 tbsp of coconut oil, ghee or butter, melted

2/3 (3.8 oz) Cup of unsalted pumpkin seeds

1 (1.75 lbs.) small organic head of cauliflower, chopped evenly into sizes or 20 oz. frozen cauliflower

INSTRUCTIONS

1. Heat the oven to 375 degrees F. Lightly roast the pumpkin seeds for 4 to 6 minutes in the oven, keep a close eye on it and remove immediately is starts to change color. Set aside to cool.

2. Pour the chopped cauliflower into casserole dish, toss with melted oil/ ghee.

3. Increase oven temperature to 400 and bake the cauliflower (covered) for 35 – 40 minutes in the oven, stirring 3 times during baking until very soft. Remove the lid once its 10 minutes to the final baking time. (You can use other methods also either by steaming or boiling).

4. Once the pumpkin seeds are cooled, pour into the food processor and grind into very fine meal.

5. Add the lemon juice, olive oil, cooked cauliflower, salt and pepper into the processor. Process until a smooth paste emerges.

6. Pour in chopped cilantro, process a little bit just to chop into smaller pieces and incorporate. Taste and add more seasonings if needed.

Spaghetti Squash With Zucchini

Prep time: minutes
Cook time: minutes
Servings: 8-10
INGREDIENTS
4 ounces of feta cheese
Pinch of freshly-ground pepper
Celtic sea salt to taste
2 cups of cooked spaghetti squash
1/2 tbsp of fresh basil (or 1/2 tsp of dried)
2-3 minced cloves garlic
1 chopped small onion
2 medium-sized zucchini or 3 small, thinly sliced (You can also use yellow summer squash)
1-3 tbsp of olive oil
INSTRUCTIONS
1. Heat one tbsp. olive oil over medium low heat in a large skillet and sauté the zucchini for 10 to 12 minutes.
2. Add the garlic and onions and sauté until zucchini is soft and onions are fragrant and translucent.
3. Add spaghetti squash and basil, stirring constantly and adding additional oil until pasta is well mixed with the squash and lightly coated with oil. Season with pepper and salt and garnish with feta cheese.

Turkey Burgers

Prep time: 10 minutes

Cook time: 10 minutes

Servings: 4

INGREDIENTS

1 tbsp of vegetable oil

½-1 tsp of white pepper

1 tsp of salt free seasoning

1 each clove garlic

1/4 cup of grated red onion

1/4 cup of panko bread crumbs

1 large egg

1 cup of grated zucchini, (about 3 small)

1 lbs of lean ground turkey

INSTRUCTIONS

1. Mix all the ingredients in a large bowl.

2. Form into about 1/2 inch thick equal patties.

3. Heat 1 tsp of vegetable oil in a large non-stick skillet over medium high heat.

4. Place the patties and turn to low heat, cook about 5 minutes on each side until browned on both sides and no longer pink in the middle.

Baked Acorn Squash

Prep Time: 10 minutes

Cook Time: 45 minutes

Servings: 3

INGREDIENTS

1/4 tsp of nutmeg

3 tbsp of pineapple, crushed

2 tsp plus 1 tbsp of unsalted butter

2 tsp of brown sugar

1 acorn squash, halved and seeded

INSTRUCTIONS

1. Heat up the oven to 400F.

2. Grease a baking pan with cooking spray and place the squash, let the cut side face up.

3. Add 1 tsp of brown sugar plus 1 tsp of butter in each of the squash half.

4. Use aluminum foil to cover squash and then place in the oven and bake approximately 30 minutes until tender.

5. Scoop out the squash from the shells, stop when the shell is about 1/4 inch thick.

6. Mix pineapple, cooked squash, nutmeg and 1 tablespoon of butter. Beat to incorporate.

7. Transfer the mixture back into shells; Place in the oven at 425 degrees for 15 minutes.

Honey Garlic Shrimp Stir Fry

Prep Time: 5 minutes

Cook Time: 7 minutes

Servings: 6

INGREDIENTS

1/4 tsp of cayenne pepper

1/4 tsp of salt

1 1/2 tbsp of lime juice

1 tbsp of honey

4 minced cloves of garlic

1 tbsp of melted butter

1 pound of shrimp shelled and deveined, rinse in cold water

INSTRUCTIONS

1. Add butter into a hot skillet, and sauté the garlic until brown.

2. Add lime juice, honey, cayenne pepper.

3. Add the shrimp, stir and cook over medium-high heat for two minutes or until pink throughout and sauce has thicken.

Serve shrimp over cauliflower rice.

Crispy Parmesan Chips

Prep Time: 70 minutes

Cook Time: 0 minutes

Servings: (6) 2 chip per serving

INGREDIENTS

1 cup of shredded parmesan cheese

1/8 tsp of salt

1/8 tsp of white pepper

¼ tsp of onion powder

¼ tsp of garlic powder

INSTRUCTIONS

1. Heat the oven to 425 F. Spray your baking pan with cooking spray, and then line the baking pan with parchment paper.

2. In a mixing bowl, mix the garlic powder, onion powder, salt, white pepper with parmesan cheese until the cheese is well coated.

3. Spoon a tablespoon of the mixture into the baking sheet, spacing about 1 inch. Press down to flatten each cheese.

4. Bake in the preheated oven for 7 to 10 minutes until completely melted. But be on the lookout, the chips can burn quickly!

5. Let cool in the baking sheet, then transfer to a serving dish.

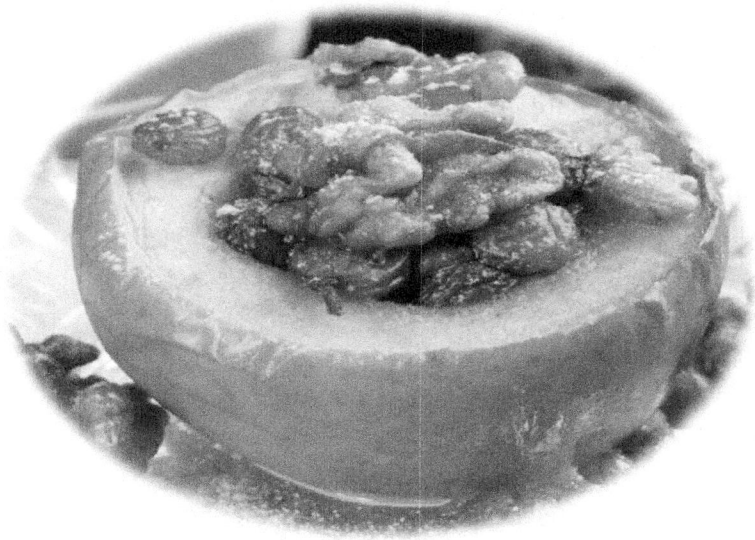

No-bake Coconut Bars

Prep Time: 40 minutes

Servings: 9

INGREDIENTS

½ cup of melted coconut oil

½ cup of sunflower butter

3 scoops of vanilla protein powder

1 tbsp of milled flaxseed

1 large ripe banana

3 tbsp of unsweetened coconut shreds

2 cups of oats

INSTRUCTIONS

1. Mash the ripe banana until the consistency is smooth. Add the remaining ingredients and mix to combine.

2. Add the mixture into a square pan, press down to level. Place pan in the freezer for about 30 minutes to firm up. Cut into squares and wrap individually.

Lettuce Wraps

Prep Time: 10 minutes

Servings: 4

INGREDIENTS

Half head butter lettuce

1 lbs of thick bacon, cut into 1" pieces

1 cup of shredded cheddar cheese

10 cherry tomatoes

INSTRUCTIONS

1. Heat a large skillet over medium heat, add bacon pieces and cook until evenly brown. Set aside.

2. Divide the cherry tomatoes into two.

3. Arrange ¼ cup of cheddar cheese on each of the lettuce leaf, top with ¼ of the bacon and ¼ of the cherry tomatoes.

4. Roll up wraps, then slice in half.

Golden Fried Apples

Prep Time: minutes

Total Time: minutes

Servings: 6- 8

INGREDIENTS

(Optional) A drizzle of honey

2 tbsp of butter or coconut oil

1/4 tsp of nutmeg (or 1/4 tsp of cinnamon but oxalate content will be higher)

6 – 8 medium Granny Smith apples, cored and cut into thin slices(peeling, optional)

INSTRUCTIONS

1. Heat the butter in a sauce pan over medium heat. Place the apples slices and sauté for few minutes until apples are tender and some of the apples are golden brown. Sprinkle top of apples with nutmeg and add spread with honey. Stir to coat with the apples.

Butternut Squash Apples

Prep Time: 20 minutes

Cook Time: 60 minutes

Servings: 8

INGREDIENTS

1 tbsp of sugar

1/4 tsp of cinnamon

3 peeled and cored medium apples or 12 ounces of applesauce

1/4 tsp of pepper

1/2 tsp of salt

1 tbsp of butter

1 10 oz bag of frozen butternut squash or 1.5 pounds of fresh butternut squash

1/4 cup of chopped pecans

INSTRUCTIONS

1. Heat-up the oven to 350 F.

2. Place the butternut squash in the microwave and cook as directions on bag instruction. OR peel and remove seeds if using butternut squash. Cut in large pieces. Boil squash for 20-30 minutes in a skillet over medium heat until tender. Drain.

3. Add the cooked squash in a medium bowl, and carefully mash some of the pieces.

4. Gently mix in the remaining ingredients into the squash.

5. Spoon squash mixture into an 8" square glass dish or 9" pie dish.

6. Place in the oven and bake at 350 F for 25-30 minutes.

Cheesy Herbs Dip

Servings: 10 servings per recipe

Low sodium, Low Potassium, Low Protein, Low Phosphorus

INGREDIENTS

½ tsp of garlic powder

½ tsp of thyme

½ tsp of basil

½ tsp of pepper

1 tbsp of green onions, minced

1 tbsp of fresh parsley, chopped

250 grams of cottage cheese 2% M.F.

250 grams of low fat cream cheese

INSTRUCTIONS

1. Mix together all ingredients in a blender or food processor

2. Place in the refrigerator to chill.

Serve with grilled tortillas or as a spread in a sandwich.

DESSERTS RECIPES

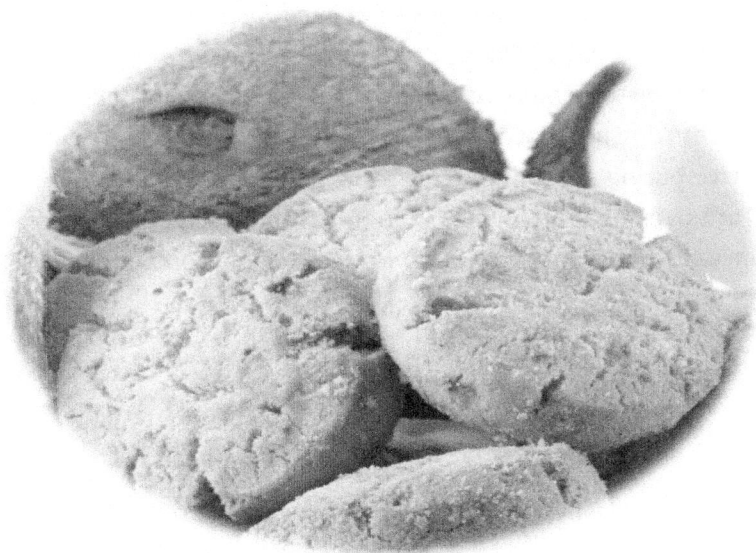

Tasty Coconut Cookies

Prep time: 5 minutes

Cook time: 9 minutes

Servings: 8

INGREDIENTS

2 tablespoons of cold butter

1 tablespoon of honey

3 tablespoons of coconut flour

INSTRUCTIONS

1. Preheat the oven to 365 F.

2. Combine the ingredients together in a food processor or blender and blend until well mixed.

3. Mould mixture into small balls, place onto a cookie baking sheet and press down to flatten.

4. Place baking sheet in the oven and bake for 9 minutes.

5. Turn oven heat off and let sit in the oven for 2 minutes. Remove from oven and transfer onto a wire rack to cool completely.

Cool Macaroons

Prep Time: 5 minutes

Cook Time: 15 minutes

Servings: 20

INGREDIENTS

Pinch of salt

1 tsp of vanilla extract

3 egg whites

2 1/2 cups of shredded unsweetened coconut

3/4 cup of raw honey

INSTRUCTIONS

1. Heat-up the oven to 350 F.

2. In a large bowl, mix together the entire ingredients with your hands or rubber spatula.

3. With wet hands shape the coconut mixture into small balls and place onto sheet pans lined with parchment paper, about an inch apart

4. Place in the oven and bake about 15 minutes until light brown.

5. Remove from the oven and let cool for at least 30 minutes on a rack before serving.

Store leftover in a covered container, can keep for 3 days.

Caramel Apple Cake

Prep time: 10 minutes

Cook time: 50 minutes

Servings: 12

INGREDIENTS

3 medium apples, (Granny Smith) peeled, cored and diced

1 box yellow cake mix or any sugar free cake mix

3/4 cup of flour

12 egg whites

1/4 cup of vegetable oil

2 tbsp of water

1/4 cup of caramel flavored syrup, sugar free or regular

INSTRUCTIONS

1. Heat up the oven to 350 F.

2. Place diced apples in the microwave on high for 6 minutes or until soft. Mash unto applesauce and allow cooling on room temperature.

3. Add flour, cake mix, caramel flavoring, apple mixture, water, vegetable oil and egg whites in a mixing bowl. Mix for 1 minute on low speed, scraping down the sides. Then Mix on medium speed for two minutes.

4. Transfer the batter into a 9 X 13 baking dish or two greased loaf pans.

5. Place in the oven and bake about for 30-45 minutes until a skewer inserted in the middle comes out clean.

6. Allow the cake to cool, then sprinkle with powdered sugar.

Pumpkin seeds Cookies

Prep Time: 5 minutes

Total Time: 5 minutes

Servings: 20

INGREDIENTS

2 tbsp of honey

1 tbsp of olive oil

1/2 tsp of xanthan gum

1/4 tsp of baking soda

1/4 tsp of cream of tartar

4 tbsp of ground linseed/flax

1/4 cup of ground pumpkin seeds

1/4 cup of brown rice flour

Water as needed

INSTRUCTIONS

1. Combine together all the dry ingredients in a bowl. Stir in honey and oil until texture resembles breadcrumbs.

2. Add water to the mixture (1 tsp. at a time) until a dough is formed.

3. Divide dough into 2 even balls, and then roll each ball out between 2 sheets of parchment paper and cut into 20 cookies.

4. Bake in oven for 3 minutes at at 374 F, check and flip for extra 1-2 mins.

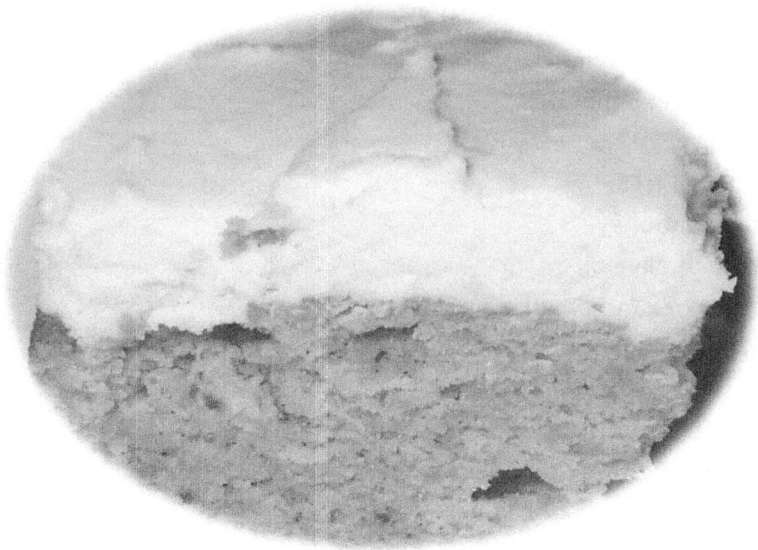

Low Oxalate Ice Cream

INGREDIENTS

5 frozen strawberries

2-3 tsp of vanilla

1/4 cup of honey

1/4 cup of coconut oil

Pinch of salt

2 egg whites (use yolks for something else)

4 eggs, yolk separated from white

INSTRUCTIONS

1. Place the loaf pan in the freezer to freeze up.

2. Whisk six eggs whites in a bowl, add salt and whisk until stiff.

3. Slowly add in the 4 yolks, (you can use the remaining 2 yolks for something else) coconut oil, strawberries, honey and vanilla. Transfer to the freezer.

Flavored Bar

Prep Time: 15 minutes

Total Time: 2hours 15 minutes

INGREDIENTS

1 14 oz. can of sweetened condensed milk

1 1/3 cups of shredded coconut

(Optional) 1 cup of chopped macadamia nuts

1 cup of butterscotch chips

1 cup of white chocolate chips

1/2 cup of unsalted butter, cut up

1.5 cups of corn flake crumbs

INSTRUCTIONS

1. Preheat your oven to 350 degrees.

2. Line the entire 13 X 9 baking sheet with parchment paper.

3. Melt butter in the microwave. Combine melted butter with cornflake crumbs and lightly mix.

4. Add cornflake crumbs mixture to the baking pan and press down a bit into a layer.

5. Layer the cornflake crumb layer with a sprinkle of chopped nuts, then a sprinkle of chocolate chips. Top with the butterscotch chips. Add milk over the top. And lastly, sprinkle top with coconut shredded.

6. Place pan in the oven and bake for 25 minutes until lightly browned. Let cool until you can handle. Lift out of pan, using the parchment to lift, slice into squares.

Raisin Oatmeal butter Cookies

Prep Time: 18 minutes

Cook Time: 13 minutes

Servings: 18 -20 cookies

INGREDIENTS

½ cup of raisins

1 ½ cups of GF rolled oats or GF quick oats

2 tbsp of brown sugar

¼ – ½ cup of sugar (to taste)

¼ tsp of salt

¼ tsp of baking soda

1 tsp of pure vanilla extract

1/3 cup of apple sauce

1/3 cup of Sunbutter

1 tbsp of warm lemon juice

¼ cup of warm water

2 tbsp of ground flax seed

INSTRUCTIONS

1. In a mixing bowl, combine together the lemon juice, ground flax and water. Set aside for about 5 to 8 minutes until mixture begin to look goopy.

2. Add vanilla, apple sauce, sunflower butter, baking soda, sugar and salt. Stir until thoroughly mixed.

3. Add the raisins plus oats and mix to combine. Let sit for 5 to 10 minutes.

4. Spoon about a tablespoons of the batter scantily onto a greased cookie sheet.

5. Bake in the oven for 11 – 13 minutes at 350 degrees until golden brown.

Cherry And Apple Chutney

Prep Time: 5 minutes

Cook Time: 15 minutes

Servings: 32 (1 Tbsp Each) servings per recipe

INGREDIENTS

1 1/2 cups of sugar

1 cup of apple cider vinegar

1 thinly sliced small red onion

1 cup of dried tart cherries

1 medium tart apple

INSTRUCTIONS

1. Cut the apples into 4 parts, core and cut into thin slices. (Skin on).

2. In a heavy saucepan, add cherries, apples, onions, sugar and vinegar.

3. Cook and keep stirring until mixture is starting to boil and sugar is dissolved.

4. Cover with the lid and cook on low heat, about 8-10 minutes until onions are soft and cherries are soft and plump.

5. Remove lid and increase to high heat, boil about 5 minutes more until the syrup around the fruit is reduced to a shiny glaze. Serve and enjoy. Leftovers can be kept in the refrigerator, covered for several days.

Blueberry cheese Pie

Prep Time: 7 minutes

Cook Time: 7 minutes

Servings: 9

INGREDIENTS

3 cups of blueberries

8 oz of tub non-dairy whipped cream

2 tsp of lemon juice

1 tsp of vanilla extract

1/4 cup of granulated sugar

8 oz of softened cream cheese

1/2 cup of melted butter, unsalted

1/4 tsp of cinnamon

2 cups of graham cracker crumbs

INSTRUCTIONS

1. Heat up oven to 375 F.

2. Combine the cinnamon, butter and cracker crumbs in a medium bowl.

3. In the base of a 9 inch baking dish, Spread and press the mixture evenly to form a crust.

4. Place in the oven and bake, about 7 minutes. Let cool.

5. Soften cream cheese with sugar using electric mixer to mix in a large bowl, until smooth.

6. Stir in lemon juice and vanilla extract and slowly mix in the whipped and then slowly mix in the blueberries.

7. Evenly spread the mixture on top the crust.

8. Allow chilling, covered in the refrigerator for up to an hour.

Butternut Squash Cake with Cream Cheese frosting

Prep Time: 10 minutes

Cook Time: 35 minutes

Servings: 12 -15

INGREDIENTS

Cream Cheese Icing

INGREDIENTS

2 tsp of pure vanilla extract

1/2 cup of pure maple syrup, grade B

1/4 cup of softened butter

16 ounces of softened cream cheese

INSTRUCTIONS

1. Mix the softened butter, syrup, softened cream cheese and vanilla with a hand mixer, until smooth.

For The Cake

1/2 cup of raisins

1 cup of maple syrup, grade B

1 cup of coconut oil, melted

1 tbsp of pure vanilla extract

1 tbsp of raw ginger, grated

10 eggs

1 tsp of salt

1 tsp of GF baking soda

2 tsp of cardamom

3/4 cup of coconut flour

3 cups of raw butternut squash, shredded (about 1 large)

INSTRUCTIONS

1. Heat the oven to 325 F. Greased a 13 X 9 inch cake pan.

2. Peel and remove seeds from the butternut squash; then shred by hand or use the shredding blade in a food processor.

3. In a small bowl, mix together the cardamom, flour, baking soda and salt.

4. Combine the coconut oil, ginger, eggs, maple syrup and vanilla in a separate bowl, beat with an electric hand mixer.

5. Gently add the dry mixture into the wet mixture and mix well.

6. Mix in the raisins and shredded squash.

7. Pour the batter into the prepared cake pan.

8. Bake in the oven at 325 F for about 35 minutes, or until a tester (toothpick or knife) you insert in the center comes out clean. Allow cake to completely cool before frosting.

Made in the USA
Monee, IL
21 October 2020

45679839R00069